INTRODUCTION TO THE COMBINED VERSI

I had no idea what to expect when I published the first Unreported Truths booklet in June.

I had a decent audience on Twitter for my arguments that governments all over the world had overreacted to the relatively minor threat Sars-Cov-2 posed. But I didn't know if anyone would want to read the details of how we count Covid deaths and the reality that most victims are very old and sick. I figured maybe a few thousand people might pay $2.99 for an ebook of what I initially called the "Essential Guide to Covid." (At the last minute I decided that title made it sound like a travel guide for backpackers and Unreported Truths would be both more accurate and punchier.)

Instead – thanks in part to Amazon, which provided priceless publicity when it tried to keep me from publishing the book – that many people bought it in the first few *hours* it was on sale. Over 150,000 people have now purchased Part 1. Parts 2 and 3, which cover the (in)effectiveness of lockdowns and masks, have sold solidly too.

More recently, the physical booklets have outsold the Kindle versions. The gap has surprised me, because the physical booklets cost twice as much. (For what it's worth, I actually make less on the booklets, because of the cost of printing and distributing them.)

The booklets haven't won because of snazzy design, either. Black print on a grey cover (Part 2 was white), simple large font, a couple of chapters. No graphics or maps or photos. To Amazon's credit, it can print and deliver lots of copies fast. But on a semi-regular basis those copies have extra blank pages or other printing mistakes.

Why, then? What's the appeal of a physical booklet that readers must wait days to receive instead of the instant gratification of a download? A reviewer for Townhall.com explained the phenomenon in a review of Part 3. In an age when Amazon and other big technology companies routinely suppress information they do not like, having a physical booklet that technology giants cannot control is comforting:

> Like a hand-written letter in the mail, there's something quaint yet quietly powerful about using print media to distribute something the powers-that-be clearly do not want the public to read...
>
> [H]olding this 39-page pamphlet in my hands and personally handing it to friends and family to read feels like a throwback to another era, something dissidents from 'establishment' thought on any topic have done since the invention of the printing press. Try 'deleting' this now, Big Tech!

A throwback indeed. During the Communist era, dissidents in the Soviet Union copied and pasted booklets with information their would-be masters wanted to censor. They called the process *samizdat*, the Russian word for "self-publishing."

But the history of protest pamphlets goes back even further in the United States – at least to Thomas Paine and "Common Sense" in 1775. Make no mistake, this series is in the tradition of those pamphlets. With a twist. My argument is for the most part fact-driven, not philosophical. Unlike Paine, I'm not trying to convince you that we all have inalienable rights and don't have to follow a king's dictates. Hopefully we can agree on that much.

Yes, I have a political goal – to convince you that lockdowns and other Covid-related governmental intrusions are for the most part a mistake. But I'm using *journalistic and scientific* means. I am offering information and data that major media outlets have failed to report and making a case they will not present. I provide links to the major documents I quote because I want you the reader to be able to judge them yourself.

In fact, I *agree* governments may sometimes be justified in taking strong measures to prevent the spread of dangerous diseases. I believe – as most public health experts did before March – that the bar for lockdowns should be very high. But very high doesn't mean impossible. If the coronavirus killed 5 or 10 percent of the people it infected, decisive steps would be justified. (And if killed 80 percent or more, as inhaled anthrax does, we would *expect* to remake society completely. Luckily anthrax cannot be spread person to person.)

But the coronavirus doesn't kill 80 percent of the people who get it. Or 10 percent. Or 5 percent. Or 1 percent. Or 0.5 percent. Worldwide, it probably kills somewhere around 0.1 or 0.15 percent of the people it infects. In other words, about 999 out of 1,000 people who get it will survive.

That fact is the *most* fundamental unreported truth about the coronavirus. It is simply far less deadly than most people understand. The risk it does pose is mostly to the extremely elderly and unwell. This fact was clear as early as March and has only become more obvious since.

But the vast majority of major media outlets and health experts have engaged in what can only be called a coordinated campaign to hide that fact. In doing so, they have driven a dangerous overreaction. Yes, the coronavirus can stress regional health-care networks because it is highly contagious indoors. But it has *never* presented major risks to society or most people.

I have spent the last nine months doing everything I can to make that case, with limited success. I'll keep trying. I have heard from too many people whose lives have been ruined by lockdowns or school closures to stop.

By its nature, journalism generally has a short shelf life. *Yesterday's news wraps tomorrow's fish,* the old saying goes. But the booklets have already turned out to be hardier than I feared they might be. Together, they have now received more than 10,000 reviews on Amazon – and they average a nearly perfect rating, higher than any other book I have ever written. Naturally, most mainstream media outlets have ignored them. But I would like to believe that when historians look back at the roots of the mass hysteria of 2020, they will find this work not entirely useless.

So, as I work on a longer book about the crisis and consider more booklets, I decided to combine Parts 1, 2, and 3 into a more attractive and durable paperback. For convenience, I have renumbered the chapters and made a handful of extremely minor copy-editing fixes. But I have not otherwise changed the original booklets. (Lately, newspapers – including my old employer The New York Times – have taken advantage of the frictionless editing the Internet offers to make secret changes to articles after publication. I think this trend is wrong, and I won't take part in it.)

Naturally, the new version will be available as an ebook too. Plenty of readers prefer the convenience and lower cost. But I can't help hoping you'll buy the physical version, and that it stays on your bookshelf long after the coronavirus and 2020 are nothing more than unpleasant memories.

Stay sane -

Alex

UNREPORTED TRUTHS ABOUT COVID-19 AND LOCKDOWNS:

PART 1:

Introduction and Death Counts and Estimates

(Published June 4, 2020)

INTRODUCTION

I'm as surprised as you are that I'm writing this booklet.

When the coronavirus first emerged in China in January, I was researching American drug policy, working on a follow-up to *Tell Your Children,* my 2019 book on the mental health risks of cannabis.

But I couldn't stop reading about the virus – officially called SARS-COV-2. On conventional and social media, the news worsened by the day. Hospitals in the 10-million-person Chinese city of Wuhan were overrun. Videos on Twitter showed people dropping dead in the street and hospitals filled with body bags. Epidemiologists and scientists predicted the coronavirus would ravage other Chinese megacities.

In mid-February, the crisis seemed to pause. But by the end of the month, the coffins were stacking up in northern Italy, and the lockdowns beginning. Meanwhile, the United States reported its first deaths, at a nursing home in Seattle.

By early March I genuinely feared the United States might face an outbreak that would kill millions of Americans and potentially destabilize the nation. I loaded up on food for our family, bought the last N95 masks I could find at the local Wal-Mart, watched the stock market plunge.

Then, on Monday, March 16, Imperial College publicly released its now-infamous research report (https://www.imperial.ac.uk/media/imperial-college/medicine/sph/ide/gida-fellowships/Imperial-College-COVID19-NPI-modelling-16-03-2020.pdf) predicting coronavirus might kill a half-million Britons and two million Americans if governments didn't act immediately to close schools and businesses.

Worse, the report forecast 1.1 million Americans and 250,000 people in the United Kingdom could die even with months of efforts to reduce the damage. Only long-term "suppression" of society – possibly until a vaccine was invented – could lower those figures meaningfully, the researchers wrote.

The Imperial College researchers weren't just any academics. They worked directly with the World Health Organization. Their forecast terrified politicians across Europe and the United States and spurred what became a near-worldwide lockdown. Yet, ironically, the Imperial College report marked the beginning of my understanding of the realities of COVID-19. It planted the seeds of my skepticism about the lockdowns and our response to the coronavirus since.

Why?

When I read the report that Monday night, I noticed a chart on page 5 showing the likelihood of death in different age ranges. The chart showed coronavirus was more than 100 times as likely to kill people over 80 than under 50. Yes, 100 times. People under 30 were at very low risk.

The information stunned me. I knew coronavirus was more dangerous to older people, of course – but I assumed young people would also face serious risks. After all, any really deadly virus could hardly spare the young or middle-aged. A century ago, the Spanish flu killed children and young adults along with the elderly.

I found myself thinking of China. Not about what *had* happened in Wuhan, but about what *hadn't* happened everywhere else. Shanghai and Beijing and other huge cities had avoided catastrophe. In early February, epidemiologists warned the

Chinese lockdowns had come too late to matter. Instead, China was already tentatively reopening, restarting factories and dropping quarantines. If the virus was so deadly, how come the Chinese – who at that point had seen it more closely than anyone else – weren't more frightened?

I came back to the Page 5 chart again and again. I found myself asking two related questions: Why wasn't the media telling the truth about the huge difference in risk by age?

And was the coronavirus really as deadly as I and everyone else believed?

Nine days later, on March 25, the lead author of the Imperial College report, professor Neil Ferguson, testified about coronavirus to a committee of the British Parliament. Ferguson calls himself an epidemiologist, though he is not a physician and his doctorate is in theoretical physics. He was testifying remotely, since he had contracted the coronavirus a week before and was in a self-imposed home quarantine. (Later, a British newspaper would break the news that Ferguson had violated his isolation to have sex with a married woman he met on OKCupid; he was forced to resign in disgrace from a scientific committee advising the British government on the epidemic. But at the time his reputation was sterling and his previous forecasting mistakes – which are legion and in some cases comical – largely forgotten.)

Ferguson's testimony to the committee received no attention in the US. American media were focused on the emerging crisis in New York City. But British newspapers reported that Ferguson had dramatically changed his predictions. He now said his new best estimate was 20,000 Britons would die from the virus even with just weeks of quarantines. Further, because the virus is far more dangerous to the elderly and people with severe health problems, more than half of those 20,000 people would probably have died in 2020 in any case, he said. (https://www.telegraph.co.uk/news/2020/03/25/two-thirds-patients-die-coronavirus-would-have-died-year-anyway/)

For the second time in just over a week, I found myself stunned. Instead of 500,000 British deaths, 20,000? Without months or years of lockdowns? In the absence of a vaccine or effective treatment? Had Ferguson just cut the Imperial College estimate by 96 percent (or 92 percent, if one used the 250,000-person death estimate)? What facts could have changed so much in just a few days? What did the change say about the accuracy of either the old or the new estimate?

And, again, why hadn't the New York Times and other American media outlets – after giving the earlier estimate so much attention – given equal prominence to the new number?

Investigative reporters have an old saw: *If your mother says she loves you, check it out.* In other words, question everything. But no one in the media seemed to be questioning anything. Instead, journalists were topping themselves with forecasts of doom. Molly Jong-Fast, an editor at the Daily Beast, told her 500,000 Twitter followers that as many as 7 percent of Americans – 23 million people – would die (https://twitter.com/mollyjongfast/status/12425081736275312 69). The Times reporter Trip Gabriel predicted the United States was "expected" to need one million ventilators, the machines that breathe for people who can't on their own (https://twitter.com/tripgabriel/status/1242979481524076544? lang=en).

Gabriel's comment was absurd on its face. Ventilators are complex machines. Training physicians and respiratory therapists to use them takes years. Thus, even if we'd suddenly built a million ventilators, hospitals couldn't possibly have put people on them. If a million people at once were about to become so gravely ill that they needed ventilators, the apocalypse was truly nigh.

My instincts as an investigative reporter took over. I had been a New York Times reporter from 1999 until 2010, but I didn't work for the Times anymore. Even if I had been working for them, I doubted they would be interested in my efforts to challenge the narrative. They were among the leaders of what I had begun to think of as "Team Apocalypse," the media outlets that – for reasons I could not fully understand – seemed committed to painting as bleak a picture of the coronavirus as possible.

I had one outlet: Twitter. At the time I only had about 10,000 followers, but I was a verified account (in Twitter lingo, a blue-check), which gave me a bit of extra credibility. And I didn't have other options to ask questions in real time. The day after Ferguson's testimony, March 26, I raised questions about his revised estimate in a series of tweets.

For better or worse, people noticed. The most notable was Elon Musk, who besides being the founder of Tesla and SpaceX has a huge Twitter audience, with tens of millions of followers. Musk and others retweeted my primary tweet challenging Ferguson, and it was viewed almost 5 million times.

Suddenly I found myself as one of the few people with any journalistic standing challenging the apocalyptic reporting that dominated media outlets like the Times. Over the next few days, I pointed out on Twitter that a model from the University of Washington used to predict hospitalizations and intensive care needs was proving hugely wrong in its forecasts – even in New York, where the problems were worst.

Within a few days, "senior officials" in the White House had begun to notice the tweets and the questions they raised, according to New York Times reporter Maggie Haberman. (https://twitter.com/maggienyt/status/1246805287627079681 ?lang=en)

Nonetheless, this view was less than popular, to say the least. Through late March and early April scorn and hate poured in, especially from my fellow media "blue checks." People wished for me to die of coronavirus, which didn't really bother me, except when they said they hoped my family would too. The fear coming out of New York City, where so many members of the media lived, was palpable.

But as the days passed, the fact that the models were profoundly overestimating the number of people who would need to be hospitalized with SARS-COV-2 became self-evident. Despite repeated revisions, the model from the University of Washington continued to fail – not after months or even weeks, but on a daily basis.

In turn, the importance of that failure became increasingly obvious to me and a handful of other skeptics. What had happened in New York City in March was not generalizable to the rest of the United States. Hospitals outside New York were mostly empty and furloughing workers. Worse, in some cases they were *shutting down* because they had so few patients – a bizarre paradox in what was supposed to be the worst epidemic since the Spanish Flu a century before. (https://www.alvareviewcourier.com/story/2020/04/10/region al/oklahoma-city-hospital-closed-amid-coronavirus-spread/62038.html)

Even in New York, the health-care system was never close to being overrun. Field hospitals built at a cost of tens of millions of dollars were dismantled; some had never seen a single patient. Navy hospital ships departed the harbor, searching in vain for new coronavirus hotspots. In late March, New York governor Andrew Cuomo had said the state might need 140,000 hospital beds and up to 40,000 ventilators. "Everybody's entitled to their own opinion, but I don't operate here on opinion. I operate on facts and on data and on numbers and on projections," Cuomo said.

https://www.syracuse.com/coronavirus/2020/03/cuomo-refutes-trump-insists-ny-needs-up-to-40000-ventilators-i-operate-on-facts.html

In the end, New York never had more than 4,000 coronavirus patients on ventilators – making Cuomo's facts and data and numbers and projections off by about tenfold.

By mid-April, it was obvious to me – and anyone who was paying attention – that the coronavirus epidemic simply was not going to be anywhere near as bad as the early predictions, and that the lockdowns were an extreme overreaction.

The failure of the models should have raised an even more crucial question: setting aside the massive economic and societal harms they'd caused, had the lockdowns even helped control the spread of the coronavirus at all?

But through April and May, major media outlets resolutely failed to ask that question. Instead, they focused nearly all their attention on COVID death counts, which rose slowly but steadily, eventually surpassing the total of 60,000 deaths initially estimated for the 2017-18 flu season.

Still, real information continued to drip out – often tucked away in scientific papers that went unnoticed, such as when a German research institute reported in mid-April that lockdowns had been broadly useless.

Yet – more than two months after they began – the lockdowns continue. Only Alaska has gone back to a pre-March normal. Even states like Georgia and Texas retain restrictions on restaurants and retailers and have not restarted their schools. Many other states, including giants like New York and Illinois, are repealing their rules slowly. In many cases they are requiring people to wear masks even in public and hinting that they will not allow schools to operate normally even in the fall.

So, yes, the coronavirus epidemic has largely ended as a medical crisis. But for now, the policies it has spawned remain educational, economic, and societal millstones. And the battles over issues such as mask-wearing, testing, contact tracing, and what to do if SARS-COV-2 regains momentum in the fall are burning hotter than ever.

Which is why I'm writing now.

I want to be clear my aims here are limited. I am not aiming here to provide a complete or even capsule history of SARS-COV-2, its initial spread in China in January, or the decisions that the United States and other countries made in February and March. For example, whether the virus emerged from a Chinese biological research laboratory is a fascinating question. Eventually we may have a definitive answer. But for now anything I write would be speculation.

Nor will I spend time making specific judgments about coronavirus treatments. For example, I won't write about the various medicines now being tested for COVID, including hydroxychloroquine. Scientists and physicians are still examining those drugs in clinical trials. Until those trials are complete, even the doctors who use them can't be sure if they are working. For me to pretend I know what might work is worse than useless.

Eventually, I may write a longer book about SARS-COV-2 (I'll have lots of competition). If and when I do, I'll try to address the broader questions – though even a moderately comprehensive account may take years to research and write. The coronavirus, and the way we responded to it, will be grist for physicians and scientists and economists and historians and journalists for many years to come.

Instead of those broader topics, I want to focus here on crucial questions that I have tried to answer – or at least raise – in my Twitter feed in the last two months, including:

How lethal is SARS-COV-2? Is it more dangerous than the flu?

Who is most at risk?

How are SARS-COV-2 deaths coded? What questions does that coding policy raise?

What are the main ways in which the coronavirus has spread? How long has it been circulating?

How many people have already been infected?

Why did the key predictive models that policymakers used when they agreed to lockdowns prove so inaccurate?

Do lockdowns slow the spread?

What is the evidence for and against lockdowns, viewed on a public health basis, without regard to their economic, educational, and societal harms?

What about those other harms? How severe are they already, and how severe might they become?

What about the mental health risks of lockdowns?

Is requiring people to wear masks in public likely to slow the spread?

We can answer some of those questions more definitively than others, but after more than four months of frantic effort by scientists, they all have been at least partly unlocked. I will provide links to the papers and data I reference so you can judge whether the sourcing backs my answers.

I am committed to following the truth and offering the most honest answers, whatever they may be. I will not sugarcoat information, whether it is positive or negative.

For that reason, I've decided to dedicate the first chapter to discussing the number of potential deaths that the coronavirus in a worst-case scenario. As you'll see, the best estimate may be that 500,000 to 600,000 Americans might die in the next year or two.

That number is much lower than the initial Imperial College estimate, and roughly in the range of people whom smoking kills every year. Still, it is far higher than even a severe seasonal flu season – and may shock some people.

However, the estimate comes with three crucial caveats.

First, it assumes that we take NO efforts to protect the elderly, especially those in nursing homes, that we develop no medicines for coronavirus, and that physicians become no better at treating it. All three of those points are clearly wrong. States are moving to protect long-term care facilities (some, like Florida, did so early on). The anti-viral medicine remdesivir has shown modest efficacy against COVID. And physicians have moved away from using ventilators aggressively, realizing that doing so can actually kill many coronavirus patients.

Second, it assumes that we will see a second wave of deaths: that the coronavirus, like the flu, will inevitably return this fall and winter. That view is the consensus among epidemiologists and scientists, and I won't challenge it (even though many epidemiologists have been badly wrong about COVID for the last three months). One counter-argument comes from Oxford University's Center for Evidence Based Medicine, which argued that "making absolute statements of certainty about 'second waves' is unwise, given the current substantial uncertainties and novelty of the evidence." (https://www.cebm.net/covid-19/covid-19-epidemic-waves/)

Third, and most importantly, the topline death figure does not account for the fact that the deaths will be heavily concentrated among the very old and sick. More than half would likely have died within weeks or months in any case, as Neil Ferguson said in his British testimony.

From any practical point of view, those deaths are unpreventable. Their timing is a function of the coronavirus, but their cause is underlying conditions such as cancer or heart disease or dementia. Meanwhile, children and young adults are at minimal risk from the virus.

Another way to look at deaths is to consider "life-years lost" – multiplying the number of deaths by the life expectancy of each person who has died. This measurement may seem cruel, but we all do it intuitively. Who would disagree that the death of a 10-year-old is harder to accept than, say, an 88-year-old? The child is only beginning her life; the man has already had his.

By the life-years standard, the coronavirus death toll appears more comparable to a single year of overdose deaths in the United States. About 70,000 people die from overdoses of opioids and other drugs every year, but they are on average far younger than those who die of coronavirus, so their overall life expectancy is similar.

Still, 600,000 deaths is a figure that can't be blinked away. As someone who has criticized lockdowns, I might seem to be hurting efforts to reopen by discussing it openly.

But it is precisely because the number appears so daunting that we must prepare for it – both practically, by monitoring hospitalizations closely and adding medical staff to hard-hit regions if necessary, and mentally, by refusing to panic again as we did in March if deaths begin to rise this fall. Going forward, we must remember the reason we locked down the United States and the rest of the world this spring was NOT to reduce coronavirus infections or deaths to zero. We have never pursued such a policy with any other respiratory virus, nor with viruses such as HIV, which until effective medicine existed killed nearly everyone who contracted it.

No, the reason we initially agreed to lockdowns was to "flatten the curve," which is a polite way of saying "to prevent coronavirus patients from collapsing our health-care system." But the system was never in danger of collapsing, lockdowns or no.

Now that fact is clear, the lockdown rationale has shifted to the much more nebulous goal of reducing coronavirus deaths at any cost – as if deaths from COVID are the only kind of deaths or societal damage that matter.

The cost of this policy shift has been enormous. In less than three months, lockdowns have done incalculable damage. They need to be lifted as soon as possible. More importantly, we must agree that we will not restore them even if coronavirus deaths rise again in the fall and winter – unless hospitals face the real risk of collapse.

The changes we have already made to protect the most vulnerable, as well as individual efforts at social distancing – which are likely to continue even without government mandates – make a large wave of deaths less likely. But one is still possible. Thus we need to be prepared and realistic.

In general, I hope that what you read will both reassure you and help you pass information to friends and neighbors who may be unnecessarily frightened. A lot of what has happened over the last couple of months has been frustrating. But I've been lucky enough to have people tell me that my Twitter feed has helped make their lives a little more manageable. I hope this booklet can do the same. I believe reality will win, and that we will escape these lockdowns and return to normal as a society. But the road has already been longer and harder than I expected. The truth is our best weapon.

Onward.

(One final note – I have decided to release this booklet in sections; putting it together has already taken longer than I expected, and I want it to be a manageable length for an online read. I do plan to offer the combined sections in a single copy, both in paper and ebook.)

1

Maybe the most important questions of all:

How lethal is SARS-COV-2?

Whom does it kill?

Are the death counts accurate – and, if not, are they over- or understated?

Estimates for the lethality of the coronavirus have varied widely since January. Early Chinese data suggested the virus might have an "infection fatality rate" as high as 1.4 – 2 percent.

A death rate in that range could mean the coronavirus might kill more than 6 million Americans, although even under the worst-case scenarios some people would not be exposed, and others might have natural immunity that would prevent them from being infected at all.

As we have learned more about the virus, estimates of its lethality have fallen. Calculating fatality rates is complex, because despite all of our testing for COVID, we still don't know how many people have been infected.

Some people who are infected may have no or mild symptoms. Even those with more severe symptoms may resist going to the hospital, then recover on their own. We have a clear view of the top of the iceberg – the serious infections that require hospitalization – but at least in the early stages of the epidemic we have to guess at the mild, hidden infections.

But to calculate the true fatality rate, we need to know the true infection rate. If 10,000 people die out of 100,000 infections,

that means the virus kills 10 percent of all the people it infects –
making it very, very dangerous. But if 10,000 people die from 10
million infections, the death rate is actually 0.1 percent – similar
to the flu.

Unfortunately, figuring out the real infection rate is very
difficult. Probably the best way is through antibody tests, which
measure how many people have already been infected and
recovered – even if they never were hospitalized or even had
symptoms. Studies in which many people in a city, state, or
even country are tested at random to see if they are currently
infected can also help. Believe it or not, so can tests of
municipal sewage. (I'll say more about all this later, in the
section on transmission rates and lockdowns.)

For now, the crucial point is this: randomized antibody tests
from all over the world have repeatedly shown many more
people have been infected with coronavirus than is revealed by
tests for active infection. Many people who are infected with
SARS-COV-2 don't even know it.

So the hidden part of the iceberg is huge. And in turn, scientists
have repeatedly reduced their estimates for how dangerous the
coronavirus might be.

The most important estimate came on May 20, when the
Centers for Disease Control reported its best estimate was that
the virus would kill 0.26 percent of people it infected, or about 1
in 400 people. (The virus would kill 0.4 percent of those who
developed symptoms. But about one out of three people would
have no symptoms at all, the CDC said.)
(https://www.cdc.gov/coronavirus/2019-ncov/hcp/planning-
scenarios.html#box.)

Similarly, a German study in April reported a fatality rate of 0.37
percent
(https://www.technologyreview.com/2020/04/09/999015/bloo

d-tests-show-15-of-people-are-now-immune-to-covid-19-in-one-town-in-germany/). A large study in April in Los Angeles predicted a death rate in the range of 0.15 to 0.3 percent.

Some estimates have been even lower. Others have been somewhat higher – especially in regions that experienced periods of severe stress on their health care systems. In New York City, for example, the death rates appear somewhat higher, possibly above 0.5 percent – though New York may be an outlier, both because it has counted deaths aggressively (more on this later) and because its hospitals seem to have used ventilators particularly aggressively.

Thus the CDC's estimate for deaths is probably the best place to begin. Using that figure along with several other papers and studies suggests the coronavirus has an infection fatality rate in the range of 0.15 percent to 0.4 percent.

In other words, SARS-COV-2 likely kills between 1 in 250 and 1 in 650 of the people whom it infects. Again, though, not everyone who is exposed will become infected. Some people do not contract the virus, perhaps because their T-cells – which help the immune system destroy invading viruses and bacteria – have already been primed by exposure to other coronaviruses. [Several other coronaviruses exist; the most common versions usually cause minor colds in the people they infect.] An early May paper in the journal Cell suggests that as many as 60 percent of people may have some preexisting immune response, though not all will necessarily be immune. (https://www.cell.com/cell/pdf/S0092-8674(20)30610-3.pdf).

The experience of outbreaks on large ships such as aircraft carriers and cruise liners also show that some people do not become infected. The best estimates are that the virus probably can infect somewhere between 50 to 70 percent of people. For example, on one French aircraft carrier, 60 percent of sailors were infected (none died and only two out of 1,074 infected sailors required intensive care).

https://www.navalnews.com/naval-news/2020/05/covid-19-aboard-french-aircraft-carrier-98-of-the-crew-now-cured/

Thus – in a worst-case scenario – if we took no steps to mitigate its spread or protect vulnerable people, a completely unchecked coronavirus might kill between 0.075 and 0.28 percent of the United States population – between 1 in 360 and 1 in 1,300 Americans.

This is **higher** than the seasonal flu in most years. Influenza is usually said to have a fatality rate among symptomatic cases of 1 in 1,000 and an overall fatality rate of around 1 in 2,000. However, influenza mutates rapidly, and its dangerousness varies year by year. The coronavirus appears far less dangerous than the Spanish flu a century ago, which was commonly said to kill 1 in 50 of the people it infected.

It appears more comparable in terms of overall mortality to the influenza epidemics of 1957 and 1968, or the British flu epidemics of the late 1990s. (Of course, the United States and United Kingdom did not only not shut down for any of those epidemics, they received little attention outside the health-care system.)

Viewed another way: On a per-person basis, the coronavirus risk is relatively small. But the United States is a big country, so on a population level the overall potential fatality numbers are eye-catching. They represent a worst-case death toll of 250,000 to 900,000 Americans. The Centers for Disease Control's estimate translates into a range of just over a half-million total coronavirus deaths, for example.

The topline coronavirus death toll is important. But arguably even more important questions are who is dying – and how long those people might have lived if the coronavirus had not killed them.

Unfortunately, those have received far less media attention, though the answers could not be clearer. Coronavirus overwhelmingly targets the very old and sick. And when they die many of those people have at most months to live.

Just how old? The median age of people killed by the coronavirus is roughly 80 to 82 worldwide. (Median represents the halfway point – half of all people are older and half younger.)

A few examples: as of May 28, the median age of the 32,000 Italians killed by COVID-19 was 81. More than 13,000 were over 80. Another 5,400 were over 90. (https://www.epicentro.iss.it/en/coronavirus/bollettino/Report-COVID-2019_28_may_2020.pdf)

In England and Wales, as of May 15, about 17,000 of the 41,000 coronavirus deaths occurred in people over 85. Another 13,000 occurred in people between 75 and 84.

(https://www.ons.gov.uk/peoplepopulationandcommunity/healthandsocialcare/conditionsanddiseases/articles/coronaviruscovid19roundup/2020-03-26)

In New York, as of May 28, almost 40 percent of the 23,700 reported deaths occurred in people over 80. (https://covid19tracker.health.ny.gov/views/NYS-COVID19-Tracker/NYSDOHCOVID-19Tracker-Fatalities?%3Aembed=yes&%3Atoolbar=no&%3Atabs=n)

In Minnesota, the median age of the 1,000 COVID deaths is almost 84. More people over 100 have died than under 50.

The pattern is the same everywhere. Extremely elderly people
are far more likely to die of SARS-COV-2 than anyone else. That
is especially true for those living in nursing homes and assisted
living facilities. Those people account for about 40 to 50 percent
of all deaths from COVID in the United States. A figure of 43
percent has been widely used. It probably understates the real
total because in some states, including New York, nursing home
residents who die in hospitals are counted as hospital deaths.

The flip side of the risk to the elderly is that younger adults and
especially teenagers and children are at extremely low risk from
SARS-COV-2. In Italy, a total of 17 people under 30 have died of
the coronavirus. In the United Kingdom, four people under 15
have died. In New York, 14 under 20 and 102 under 30.

Worldwide, it is almost certain that more people **over the age
of 100** than **under 30** have died of SARS-COV-2. Many more
children die of influenza than coronavirus; in the 2019-20 flu
season, the Centers for Disease Control received about 180
reports of pediatric flu deaths. It has received 19 reports of
coronavirus deaths in children under 15 so far.

This profound difference in risk by age has been obvious at least
since mid-March, as the Imperial College report showed. It may
only have grown since then, in part because misguided
government policies in many states and some European
countries needlessly exposed many nursing home residents to
the coronavirus.

But most people have no idea how large the gap might be, because public health authorities and lawmakers have rarely discussed it honestly. To hide the reality, authorities often refer to the age distribution of coronavirus "cases." For example, Dr. Judith Malmgren, a Washington state epidemiologist, said on May 30 (!), "We need to make it clear that it's an equal opportunity disease." She cited the growth in "cases" in people under 40.

https://www.king5.com/article/news/health/coronavirus/seattle-epidemiologist-concerned-about-spike-of-coronavirus-in-those-under-40/281-1845991d-a1f0-4530-932a-cb29ae06be7f)

But a "case" of coronavirus refers only to a positive test result showing someone has been infected. It does not mean that a person will become sick – much less that he or she will be hospitalized, need intensive care, or die. Thus discussing the age distribution of infections, while technically not untruthful, is extremely misleading.

Major media outlets like the Times and Washington Post have gone the other way, focusing enormous attention on the literal handful of cases where children or young adults may have died from coronavirus. On Twitter, reporters go further. A Washington Post reporter tweeted on May 28, "Who among us today will be dead by next month? Your cashier at the grocery store? Your best friend? Your child?"

https://twitter.com/kemettler/status/1266000325942685697

Worst of all, as it has become obvious that active infections are generally harmless to kids or young adults, media outlets and public health authorities have highlighted the potential for very rare post-infection inflammatory and immune syndromes that cause heart damage or even kill children. Other infections are also known to cause such syndromes, so the fact that SARS-COV-2 might should not be shocking. Yet the media has treated the possibility as unprecedented rather than putting it in context.

As a father, I understand why parents might be worried. But from everything we have learned in the last few months, the coronavirus is less dangerous to children than the flu, much less other common threats to kids including car accidents, drownings – and child abuse. (I'll discuss this issue more in a later booklet when in the section on schools and school reopenings.)

The shockingly wide age differential of coronavirus deaths has another major consequence – it makes properly counting and attributing deaths to the virus much more difficult.

The United States and other countries count coronavirus deaths extremely aggressively. On March 24, the Centers for Disease Control issued new guidelines for reporting coronavirus deaths, saying explicitly that "the rules for coding and selection of the underlying cause of death are expected to result in COVID19 (sic) being the underlying cause more often than not." Notably, the CDC did not require a positive coronavirus test for physicians, coroners, or health departments to find that the virus had caused the death.

"Should 'COVID-19' be reported on the death certificate only with a confirmed test? [No], COVID-19 should be reported on the death certificate for all decedents where the disease caused or **is assumed to have caused or contributed to death.** [Emphasis added.]"

https://www.cdc.gov/nchs/data/nvss/coronavirus/Alert-2-New-ICD-code-introduced-for-COVID-19-deaths.pdf

Many states assume that anyone with a positive coronavirus test has died from the disease, no matter what their actual cause of death. As the director of the Illinois Department of Public Health explained in April, "If you were in hospice and had already been given a few weeks to live, and then you were also found to have COVID, that would be counted as a COVID death. It means technically even if you died of a clear alternate cause, but you had COVID at the same time, it's still listed as a COVID death."

https://week.com/2020/04/20/idph-director-explains-how-covid-deaths-are-classified/

The anomalies extend past deaths of hospice patients. For example, Washington state reported on May 21 it had included five people who had died of gunshots in its total of roughly 1,000 coronavirus deaths.
(https://www.clarkcountytoday.com/news/washington-department-of-health-clarifies-covid-19-death-numbers/)

Further, to make sure they don't miss any potential cases, some states match databases of deaths of people who have died with those who had positive coronavirus test results – and add anyone with a positive test result to their counts, even if there was no initial finding that coronavirus caused the death.
(https://jtv.tv/michigan-reports-263-coronavirus-cases-today-state-total-now-56884/)

Just how many "gunshot wound"-type deaths are in the COVID counts? We cannot be sure, because most states have not disclosed them. Colorado is an exception. It reports both "deaths among people with COVID-19" and "deaths from people who died from COVID-19."

As of June 2, Colorado reported 1,474 "deaths among cases" but 1,228 "deaths due to COVID-19," a gap of roughly 17 percent. https://covid19.colorado.gov/data/case-data

(The widely watched "worldometers.info" Website uses the higher figure; also, 804 of the "deaths among cases" occurred in people over 80, while 18 occurred in people under 40.) If the same gap applies nationally, almost 20,000 of the deaths that have been attributed to the coronavirus have at most a tenuous connection to it.

I don't mean to imply here that COVID-19 is not lethal or that most deaths listed as COVID-19 in the United States are not in some way related to the virus. The bubble of deaths in New York City in March and April is inarguable. Roughly 32,000 people died in the city over an eight-week period, about four times as many as in a normal spring. About 14,000 of those deaths were definitely COVID-related and another 5,000 were probably COVID-related.
https://www.cdc.gov/mmwr/volumes/69/wr/mm6919e5.htm

But major media outlets have repeatedly tried to make the case that somehow the United States has sharply undercounted coronavirus deaths. The fact that a significant fraction of deaths already listed as caused coronavirus are in fact "deaths among cases" strongly suggests otherwise.

An even more serious and ultimately insoluble problem in the count comes not from the coding of some deaths that are clearly unrelated to the virus as COVID-related, but because the vast majority of people who die after becoming infected with coronavirus are old and unwell. In these cases, the distinction between dying WITH coronavirus as opposed to FROM coronavirus can be nearly impossible to make.

Determining the cause of death can be a messy process. Coroners and health authorities must frequently balance an underlying illness with the event that specifically killed someone. Sometimes doing so is easy. An apparently healthy 55-year-old man who dies of a heart attack caused by a clot in his artery has died of coronary artery disease. But what if the man has diabetes, which can cause heart problems? Should the death be attributed to diabetes or heart disease?

Or what if the man drinks too much, drives his car into a tree, and bleeds to death before he can be rescued? His immediate cause of death is the hemorrhage. The accident caused the hemorrhage. But most people would agree the real cause of death in this case is alcohol abuse.

In those examples, at least, cause and effect is clear. But for contagious illnesses that mainly kill people already near death from serious underlying conditions, sorting out the "real" cause of death may be impossible.

A 2012 Canadian Broadcasting Corporation article on estimates for flu deaths highlighted this issue. Canada reports up to 8,000 deaths from influenza every year, the equivalent of more than 70,000 in the United States. But as the article noted, "Death can be complicated. If someone already extremely fragile with heart or lung disease is tipped over the edge with a flu infection, is that a flu death, or a heart death or a lung death? Which database gets to claim it?"
https://www.cbc.ca/news/health/flu-deaths-reality-check-1.1127442

Coronavirus targets people at the end of their lives even more aggressively than the flu, so the issue is even more serious. Beside Neil Ferguson's testimony in March, the fact that so many coronavirus deaths occur in nursing home patients is strong evidence that many victims had only weeks or months to live.

By the time they come to nursing homes, most people are very frail. A 2010 study in the Journal of the American Geriatrics Society found that half of all people admitted to nursing homes died within five months of admission (though the average length of stay was longer, because a fraction of residents lived several years after admission).
https://onlinelibrary.wiley.com/doi/abs/10.1111/j.1532-5415.2010.03005.x

Thus, over the course of a year or two, the coronavirus is likely to have little if any impact on the overall number of Americans who die, **even if the worst-case estimates for overall mortality are correct.** If 600,000 people die of coronavirus by the time everyone is exposed to it, but two-thirds of them would have died anyway from other illnesses, the "excess" mortality from coronavirus – people who would not have died during that period – would be 200,000 people.

But almost 6 million people die every two years in the United States. Thus 200,000 deaths would represent an increase in mortality of a little over 3 percent for the entire nation. Two hundred thousand extra deaths also equals about the same number of people who die from alcohol abuse over a two-year period, or from overdoses over a three-year-period.

Yes, coronavirus kills.

It's not alone.

UNREPORTED TRUTHS ABOUT COVID-19 AND LOCKDOWNS:

PART 2:

Update and Examinations of Lockdowns as a Strategy

(Published August 3, 2020)

2

Welcome to the second installment of "Unreported Truths."

This section will focus on the evidence lockdowns do - or don't - reduce the spread of the coronavirus. I also will examine the failure of the models that forecast virus patients would overrun hospitals. Their erroneous predictions play a crucial role in explaining whether lockdowns are effective.

But first, some background.

I've had a strange few weeks. Maybe you have too.

On Wednesday, June 3, I finished editing Part 1 of "Unreported Truths," about coronavirus death counts. I decided to publish the booklet through Amazon's self-publishing platform, Kindle Direct Publishing. I'd written twice for an Amazon program called "Kindle Singles," where the company publishes pieces from professional writers. So, although I knew Unreported Truths might anger some people in the media, I figured Amazon would be fine with it.

After all, Amazon sells "Mein Kampf" and "The Anarchist's Cookbook" and "Bestiality and Zoophilia: Sexual Relations with Animals." As it should. Amazon should not judge the books on its digital shelves, except in very rare cases where they offer specific advice on criminal behavior. Amazon seems to agree it should err on the side of making books available. In a statement in April, a company spokesman wrote that "As a bookseller, we believe that providing access to the written word is important, [including] books that some may find objectionable."
https://www.propublica.org/article/the-hate-store-amazons-self-publishing-arm-is-a-haven-for-white-supremacists

I also knew nothing in Part 1 could be considered a conspiracy theory. Nearly all the data in it comes from published scientific papers and official government sources. So when I uploaded Part 1 to the Kindle Direct site on Wednesday night, I figured I'd see it for sale on Amazon the next morning.

Wrong. When I checked KDP in the morning I found the book, which had been listed as being "In Review," had been returned to "Draft" status. Then Amazon emailed me:

> Your book does not comply with our guidelines. As a result we are not offering your book for sale... **Please consider removing references to COVID-19 for this book.** [Emphasis added.]

Obviously, I would have a tough time removing references to COVID-19 in a book about COVID-19.

I was shocked. Besides the company's supposed commitment to free speech, Amazon had benefitted hugely from the coronavirus lockdowns, which had forced many competitors to close. Its stock was at an all-time high, giving it an astronomical value, more than $1 trillion. (It has risen even higher since.) Under the circumstances, I thought Amazon had a special obligation to let people offer criticisms of the lockdowns. Apparently not.

I considered making the book available through my Website, but Amazon has a huge share of both the e-and physical book markets. And Amazon can sell, print, and deliver books faster than anyone else. Traditional publishers told me they would need up to a month to get the pamphlet out. Amazon could make copies available in days. I *needed* access to Amazon's audience.

I knew trying to force Amazon's hand would probably fail. The company is notoriously unresponsive to criticism. Still, I figured making noise couldn't hurt. What could Amazon do, ban the book? It already had. I went to Twitter, where my contrarian stance on lockdowns had gained me more than 100,000 followers. (Okay, that number was not even 0.2 percent as many as Kim Kardashian had, but I hoped it still might be enough to help a little.)

My heartfelt if less than eloquent plea: "Oh fuck me. I can't believe it. They censored it – " above a screenshot of the Amazon rejection email.

A number of conservative writers quickly spoke up against Amazon's censorship. So did a few on the left, notably Glenn Greenwald of The Intercept. Greenwald wrote that although he disliked my views on Covid, "book banning by corporate tech giants is a far worse danger than whatever threats [Unreported Truths] supposedly presents."

But reporters at traditional media outlets – including friends at The New York Times, *where I had worked for a decade* – mostly stayed quiet. Their silence baffled and disheartened me. Some said explicitly Amazon's audience simply shouldn't have the chance to see the booklet – a view that cuts against every idea of intellectual freedom.

By 1 p.m., I was worried. I figured if I couldn't get Amazon to pay attention by the end of the day, I might have to distribute the book myself.

Then Elon Musk stepped up.

Again.

Musk and I have still never met or even had a phone call. Maybe we never will. But if we do, I will buy him a beer (not that he needs me to buy him a beer). In the unlikely event you haven't heard of Musk, he's the chief executive of Tesla and SpaceX and has tens of millions of followers on Twitter. He is unafraid to speak his mind, and he views the lockdowns as a catastrophic mistake. He'd retweeted me before, and we had been in touch over text sporadically since early May.

I told Musk what had happened. Just before 2 p.m., he spoke up, as only he can – posting below my original tweet, "This is insane." He followed up with a second tweet, "Time to break up Amazon. Monopolies are wrong."

Musk's comments put a spotlight on Amazon's censorship. The Wall Street Journal, CNBC, and even the Washington Post – which Bezos owns – wrote articles. And someone at Amazon got the message. At 2:59 p.m., 65 minutes after Musk's tweet, I received an email from "Kindle Direct Publishing – Executive Customer Relations" telling me Amazon would publish Part 1.

Maybe Amazon would have backed down anyway. I don't know. But Musk's throwdown surely sped the process. (Amazon told reporters it had banned "Unreported Truths" in error, but it never said so to me. And it continues to ban COVID-19 books. As far as I can tell, the only error it made was censoring someone with a big enough megaphone to fight back.)

The kicker to the story came that night, after I appeared on Fox News and One America News to talk about the censorship and the booklet. I checked my Amazon sales page and found that over the course of an hour the book had sold almost *10,000* digital copies – more than two every second. By midnight it had sold 26,000. It briefly hit #1 in the Kindle Store. It has now sold more than 130,000 paper and ebook copies worldwide.

In other words, Amazon's censorship almost certainly gave "Unreported Truths" a boost. But though I was lucky, censorship by big technology companies is a growing problem. Most people who get banned aren't going to have Elon Musk to speak for them.

Meanwhile, the United States was on fire.

Through early June, the death of George Floyd sparked the most serious race-related demonstrations since the Rodney King riots of 1992. Media outlets pivoted to full-time coverage of the protests. By day, protesters filled Minneapolis, New York and other cities. By night, rioters looted stores.

The anger was real and understandable. But I assumed – wrongly, as it turned out – that the protest coverage meant the media's coronavirus hysteria was over.

The reason was simple.

The epidemic was fading across most of the world. European countries had reopened without problems. In the United States, southern states had begun to reopen more than a month earlier – Georgia on April 24, Texas not long after – without much trouble. Even in the Northeast, the hardest-hit region, states were edging towards partial reopenings. Hospitals were closing COVID-specific units and instead getting back into the business of elective surgeries and other ordinary health care.

Newspapers and cable networks were reduced to hyping case counts in countries like Peru, or writing speculative articles about potential post-infection syndromes. The most troubling example came in May, as reporters focused on a disease in children that looked very much like Kawasaki disease, which can lead to serious heart problems in kids. The New York Times led the way, writing more than a dozen articles in May. Its headlines quickly moved from claiming the illness might be "related to" coronavirus to calling it a "baffling virus syndrome."

https://www.nytimes.com/2020/05/13/health/coronavirus-children-kawasaki-pmis.html

https://www.nytimes.com/2020/05/05/nyregion/kawasaki-disease-coronavirus.html

Never mind that the syndrome appeared very rare and showed up in some kids who had not even had coronavirus infections. Never mind that the official British Kawasaki disease society repeatedly discounted the link. On May 15, the society wrote, "With continuing sensationalist press pieces causing deep worry for families, we wanted to share another paper... Children are unlikely to be seriously affected by Covid-19 infection."
https://www.societi.org.uk/kawasaki-disease-covid-19/pims-ts/

And never mind that even in serious cases of the inflammatory syndrome, most children recovered quickly after steroids or other immuno-suppressive therapy. As a Texas pediatric infectious disease expert told a television station in Austin, "'In general, most of these kids do fine.'" Which didn't stop the station from headlining its June 3 story, "Deadly illness in children linked to COVID-19 confirmed in Austin hospital."

https://www.kvue.com/article/news/health/coronavirus/multisystem-inflammatory-syndrome-dell-childrens-austin-coronavirus/269-ef12525f-213c-437a-ad9a-094f422c2f99

For months, I had referred to articles hyping the dangers of Covid as "panic porn" (and people writing them as members of "Team Apocalypse"). The Kawasaki articles were worse, frightening parents based on the thinnest possible science. I called them "kiddie panic porn," an ugly name for an ugly media game.

Yet the stories also hinted at the media's desperation to find bad news as the epidemic waned. Thus when the Floyd protests exploded I imagined the media would move away from Covid doomsaying.

I was wrong.

Since mid-June the number of positive tests for Sars-COV-2 has surged across the Sunbelt. In Florida, for example, daily positive tests rose 15-fold over a three-week period – from 617 on June 3 to more than 9,500 on June 27. Since then they have risen still further.

Many factors, both real and testing-related, are driving the rise. Restaurants are open. Voluntary social distancing has relaxed. Hot summer weather has driven people inside and increased reliance on air conditioning, which may help spread the virus. The Floyd protests and migration from Mexico may also have played a role, though those factors are more speculative.

Meanwhile, testing has skyrocketed. Some employers are requiring tests before employees can return to work. Hospitals are testing everyone who comes in for elective surgeries. The result has been a huge surge in positive tests, which the media insists on calling "cases." But using the word "case" implies someone has a clinically significant illness – that they are sick enough to need hospitalization or at least medical attention. In fact, many people infected with the coronavirus do not even know they have it, especially if they are under 50 and in decent health. They most often have either no symptoms at all or a low fever or cough, symptoms indistinguishable from a bad cold or mild flu.

Thus the increase in positive tests has far outstripped any increase in hospitalizations, intensive care admissions, ventilator use, or deaths. Every death – from Covid or any cause – is a tragedy. But for now coronavirus deaths remain significantly lower than they were in the Northeast in March and April. And we have every reason to think that they will stay that way. The vast majority of the new cases are in people under 60, who are at much lower risk. And since mid- to late July, hospitalizations have declined sharply in Arizona, Texas, and Florida – the states that led the increase.

Unfortunately, the media remains as devoted to hysteria today as in March. And the Sunbelt spike has given journalists new fuel for the panic. We are hurtling towards a fall without normal schools, while lockdowns are starting again. On July 13, California governor Gavin Newsom once again closed bars, gyms, indoor restaurant service, houses of worship, and other services.

California has about 40 million people. Since the epidemic began almost five months ago, the state has had about 9,000 deaths from the virus, *none* in anyone under 18. That's correct: Not one person under the age of 18 has died in the largest American state from Sars-Cov-2. Yet California's economy and society remain crippled.

Two big media-fed misrepresentations – I won't call them lies – work in concert to drive our policies.

First, the media has hidden the reality that anyone who is not extremely elderly or sick has a miniscule risk of dying from the coronavirus. In Part 1, I offered the real numbers and risks, based on the best government data. And since Part 1 was published, even more studies have emerged. A new Swedish government report puts the risk of death from Sars-Cov-2 at 1 in

10,000 for everyone under 50 – including those who have chronic conditions.

And in a talk on July 14, Dr. Robert Redfield, the director of the Centers for Disease Control, put the risk of deaths in children under 18 at 1 in 1 million. https://www.buckinstitute.org/covid-webinar-series-transcript-robert-redfield-md/ Major media outlets simply ignore this data.

But the media's *other* distortions are arguably even more important. Beginning in March, news outlets demanded lockdowns and lauded the public health experts who pressed for them. The few governors who resisted faced enormous pressure. A typical New York Times article from early April was headlined, "Holdout States Resist Calls for Stay-at-Home Orders: 'What Are You Waiting For?'" (https://www.nytimes.com/2020/04/03/us/coronavirus-states-without-stay-home.html)

The scrutiny extended to entire nations, such as Sweden. (https://www.cnn.com/2020/04/28/europe/sweden-coronavirus-lockdown-strategy-intl/index.html)

What went all-but-unnoticed in the push for lockdowns was the fact that major public health organizations had for decades *rejected* them as a potential solution to epidemics. In just the last three years, the Centers for Disease Control and the World Health Organization have published new epidemic planning manuals with specific recommendations about what to do if respiratory viruses hit.

The CDC published its guide in 2017, while the WHO's is even more recent and detailed. (https://www.cdc.gov/mmwr/volumes/66/rr/rr6601a1.htm) (https://apps.who.int/iris/bitstream/handle/10665/329438/978

[9241516839-eng.pdf?ua=1](9241516839-eng.pdf?ua=1)) Dozens of scientists and physicians worked on the WHO's guidelines, reviewing laboratory studies, clinical trials, and real-world evidence. The manual runs 91 pages, plus a 125-page annex with the details of the "literature reviews" used to make the recommendations. (https://apps.who.int/iris/bitstream/handle/10665/329439/WHO-WHE-IHM-GIP-2019.1-eng.pdf?ua=1)

The CDC and WHO manuals don't mention Sars-Cov-2, of course. It didn't exist when they were written. They focus on influenza epidemics. But the flu and the coronavirus are both respiratory viruses, and they are similarly infectious. So the recommendations in them should apply broadly to Sars-Cov-2. (The coronavirus is somewhat more lethal than the average flu strain but *less* lethal than some strains the WHO report anticipates.)

What's so striking about the manuals is how *little* they find effective. Even when they make recommendations – for handwashing, say, or "respiratory etiquette" (a fancy way to say "coughing into your elbow") – they acknowledge little evidence supports them. The endorsements are often made on the basis that interventions are "acceptable," "feasible," and have few "resource implications."

In other words, people can be taught to cough into their elbows and will do so without complaining. So let them try. It can't hurt. This theory extends at least partway to masks. (I'll come back to masks in a future booklet. Despite the lack of evidence for them, they have become uniquely important symbolically as a way for the media and politicians to shame people who challenge the official narrative that Sars-Cov-2 is an extraordinarily dangerous disease.)

What about lockdowns?

Both the CDC and WHO found little reason to recommend them. The 2017 CDC planner did not even mention widespread workplace closings. It discussed school closings only as a temporary measure during "severe, very severe, or extreme pandemics."

Meanwhile, the WHO report also highlighted concerns about the costs of lockdowns, noting, in language only a bureaucrat could love, that "workplace measures and closures could affect the economy and productivity of a society." It "conditionally" recommended minor measures such as "staggering shifts, and loosening policies for sick leave." It added that "workplace closure should be a last step only considered in extraordinarily severe epidemics and pandemics" – such as Spanish flu-style outbreaks that might kill "millions" of people. In other words, not the coronavirus.

Yet when Sars-Cov-2 arrived in force in Europe and the United States in March, public health authorities ignored their own cautious advice. They played a frenzied tune that the media amplified loudly enough to drown out any competing voices.

In a matter of days, dozens of countries that supposedly valued individual rights and democratic freedoms had jumped into an experiment in state control unlike any since at least World War 2.

And the lockdowns began.

3

Lockdowns, then

In theory, lockdowns can slow or even stop epidemics.

In theory.

Understanding what lockdowns actually *are* is crucial. Media outlets often use the terms lockdown, quarantine, and social distancing interchangeably. But to public health experts they are very different. Scientists use the term "quarantine" to describe confining people exposed to someone else with an infectious disease. Those quarantined people aren't even necessarily sick, but they might be. The person who actually has the disease is properly said to be not quarantined but "isolated."

A lockdown is a broader response, perhaps more accurately described as a "mass quarantine," covering a community, state, or even country. It can include canceling public gatherings like sporting events and closing schools or workplaces. In a worst-case scenario, it can even extend to ordering everyone to stay at home. It may be enforced by a national border closure or "cordon sanitaire," a police or military-enforced boundary around a region to prevent anyone from entering or exiting.

In contrast, the phrase "social distancing" generally refers to *voluntary* measures that governments encourage but don't require, like working from home. But – confusingly – journalists and even public health experts sometimes use "social distancing" as an umbrella term to include mandatory measures.

Isolation. Home quarantine. Mass quarantine. Cordon sanitaire. "Safer-at-home." "Stay-at-home." Workplace closures. Staggered shifts. Telecommuting. Essential workers. School dismissals. School closures. Lockdowns. Mitigation. Suppression. The menu of terms is in its own way telling, evidence of the choices governments must make as epidemics spread.

Of all those choices, mass lockdowns are the most powerful and disruptive.

They are also the most seductive for policymakers, at least at first, because they seem so certain to work. Like influenza, Sars-Cov-2 is a respiratory virus transmitted through relatively large droplets of virus-riddled saliva and phlegm as well as smaller particles of raw virus – so-called droplet and airborne transmission. The droplets typically stay afloat only a few feet before falling to the ground, though the airborne particles can remain aloft for longer. Flu and coronavirus can also be passed through "fomites," viral particles people pick up by touching contaminated surfaces.

Keep people far enough away from each other, and all those "vectors" of transmission should be reduced, if not eliminated entirely.

In theory.

Scientists use one simple but crucial number to determine how fast an epidemic is spreading. They call it the reproduction number, or R. It measures the number of people a newly sick person infects in turn. If R is 1, each infected person infects on average *one* other person before losing the ability to pass the virus along. If R is greater than 1, an epidemic is growing. If it is less than 1, the epidemic is dying out.

A famous shampoo ad called "And They Told Two Friends" illustrates the principle: 1 becomes 2 becomes 4 becomes 8 becomes 16 becomes 32... until everyone in the world is using Faberge shampoo. https://retroist.com/and-they-told-two-friends-how-faberge-organics-shampoo-explained-virality/

Small differences in R can make huge differences to how quickly an epidemic spreads. That is especially true in the case of respiratory viruses, which have short transmission cycles. (In other words, they make people sick quickly, but those people are infectious for only a few days.)

For example, if each person infects two more over the course of a five-day transmission cycle, a single infection will spread to more than 100 people in a month. But if each person infects three others, then a single infection will become more than 700 in a month.

But R can change dramatically and quickly, and it does not depend solely on the virus itself. Transmissibility varies over time and from place to place. Many factors can change it, both natural and human-controlled. For example, influenza viruses typically don't do well in hot weather or strong sunlight, which is why flu season typically runs from October to March. Population density is another obvious factor. The higher it is, the better chance the virus has to jump from person to person. Viruses will mutate on their own, too. In general, mutations that make the virus more transmissible but *less* dangerous to its hosts will help the virus survive better over time.

The goal of a lockdown is to reduce R – to slow the transmission rate. Ideally, a lockdown would cut R below 1, so the epidemic shrinks instead of grows. But even a lockdown that merely *slows* the growth of an epidemic – reducing R from 3 to 2, for example – can help, by reducing strain on hospitals.

When policymakers use the phrase "flatten the curve," that's what they really mean. People will still be infected, and some will still die. But the disease will spread over a longer period. So hospitals will function more normally, including continuing to treat sick people who *don't* have the virus.

Imagine a theoretically complete lockdown. Everyone must stay at home for 90 days, no matter what. Get sick? Too bad, you stay home. Need to work? Too bad, you stay home. Drones deliver food and medicine. Anyone caught outside is immediately returned home (or, in the truly dystopian version of this story, shot). Thus the virus can only spread within people living in the same house, or maybe apartment buildings with shared ventilation systems. Everyone who gets it will either recover or die by the time the lockdown ends.

Eureka, no more virus.

Obviously, even this vastly oversimplified version of the "perfect" lockdown has holes. What if the virus survives in the same animal hosts where it hid before it jumped to people? What if some people are still sick at the end? What if the virus somehow remains dormant in some people until the lockdown is over? A little-known incident at a British Antarctic base more than 50 years ago suggests just how hard suppressing respiratory viruses can be.

In 1969, six researchers at the base developed moderate to severe cold symptoms. What made the incident so fascinating was that they got sick in the middle of the Antarctic winter, after they had been isolated from all human contact for *17 weeks straight*.
(https://www.ncbi.nlm.nih.gov/pmc/articles/PMC2130424/?page=10)

"The symptoms occurring in six of 12 men were totally unexpected," scientists wrote in a 1973 paper in what at the time was called *The Journal of Hygiene* (today it is known as *Epidemiology and Infection,* a name change that neatly captures the importance of cleanliness in slowing disease). If viruses can survive winter in Antarctica, what chance does even the strictest lockdown have?

In reality, we'll never know. Because in reality, the technology to enable such a stringent lockdown doesn't exist. Drones and robots can't farm or deliver food without human help. Unless the military plans to deliver rations to everyone, private food chains must keep running. Doctors and nurses have to work. So do power plant and communications workers, prison guards and police officers. And of course scientists to monitor the virus and work on treatments.

In a modern society, the list of essential workers rises fast. Outside of dystopian science-fiction thrillers, lockdowns can *never* be complete, or even close.

In democratic nations like the United States, the obstacles to a hard lockdown are even higher. Efforts to force people to stay inside are legally problematic. Governors must instead rely on fear and public pressure. But people will resist – to protect their rights, out of boredom, or because they need to work.

Thus American lockdowns focus less on police enforcement and more on closing businesses, schools, parks, entertainment venues like movie theaters, and government offices. When there's nowhere to go except grocery stores and Wal-Mart, many people will decide leaving their houses is not worth the trouble.

How many people will stay in and how many go out? The answer depends in part on how strictly governments enforce their rules. The lockdown China imposed on Hubei province in January was far stricter than even the strictest American lockdowns, with European countries in the middle. French

authorities imposed almost a million fines, averaging more than $150, in the first month of that country's lockdown.
(https://www.thelocal.fr/20200423/french-police-hand-out-over-900000-in-lockdown-fines-including-to-holiday-home-owners)

But under any circumstances, lockdowns reduce contact between strangers, possibly by as much as 75 percent.

So in March, as the Sars-Cov-2 epidemic jumped to Europe and the United States, epidemiologists and public health experts told governments to lock down – fast and hard. Not just mass gatherings, but schools, offices, malls, even parks and beaches. To do anything less would be to sentence millions of people to death, the experts said.

Most infamously, the Imperial College London report of March 16 – written by researchers who were working with the World Health Organization – predicted more than 2 million American coronavirus deaths without immediate action. It called for a policy of what Professor Neil Ferguson, the report's lead author, termed "suppression":

> [S]uppression will minimally require a combination of social distancing of the entire population, home isolation of cases and household quarantine of their family members. This may need to be supplemented by school and university closures...

(https://www.imperial.ac.uk/media/imperial-college/medicine/sph/ide/gida-fellowships/Imperial-College-COVID19-NPI-modelling-16-03-2020.pdf)

(Of course, Professor Ferguson exempted himself from his mandate. Two weeks after the report came out, as the entire United Kingdom had locked down, and *while Ferguson himself was still supposed to be self-isolating after contracting the coronavirus,* he had an affair with a married woman who traveled across London to meet him.)

The stunning impact of the Imperial College report made Ferguson arguably the most important public health expert in the world. Yet he was neither physician nor virologist. His PhD was in theoretical physics, arguments about the structure of the universe that are something close to pure math.

But he and the other Imperial College researchers appeared to believe a handful of relatively simple equations would predict the coronavirus epidemic. To be correct, the modelers would have to understand not only how the virus spread but the complex behavioral changes lockdowns would inevitably produce. Yet the models are hardly based on *any* real data about either spread *or* lockdowns.

At their core, these models are simply software programs designed to simulate reality, based on the assumptions that the person who creates them inputs into them. They are as realistic as a game of SimCity, though less colorful.

Nonetheless, Ferguson's model produced highly precise answers. Lockdowns could reduce coronavirus deaths 95 percent or more if they continued until a vaccine was developed. Ferguson and his team even offered different death projections based on the severity of the lockdowns and benchmarks used to lift and reinstate them.

These details gave the Imperial College model an undeserved sense of certainty and reliability. In this sense, they were like other mathematical simulations of real-world events – like the ones that assumed housing prices could never collapse across the entire United States at once and thus helped cause banks in 2006 and 2007 to miss the real-estate and financial crisis they were fueling.

But for all the complexity of his equations, Ferguson really offered nothing more than an updated version of the original frightened rationale for the quarantines European city-states had imposed during the Black Death seven centuries earlier: *Keep strangers away and we'll be safe.*

The idea of using widespread lockdowns to slow epidemics took off in 2006, as The New York Times reported in April:

> Fourteen years ago, two federal government doctors, Richard Hatchett and Carter Mecher, met with a colleague at a burger joint in suburban Washington for a final review of a proposal they knew would be treated like a piñata: telling Americans to stay home from work and school the next time the country was hit by a deadly pandemic.
>
> When they presented their plan not long after, it was met with skepticism and a degree of ridicule by senior officials...

(To be clear, the Times was *lauding* Drs. Hatchett and Mecher and their work justifying lockdowns. https://www.nytimes.com/2020/04/22/us/politics/social-distancing-coronavirus.html)

After a flu scare in 2005, then-President George W. Bush asked scientists for research on slowing epidemics. Dr. Mecher, an internist at the Department of Veterans Affairs, connected with Robert Glass, a computer scientist at Sandia National Laboratories. For a science project, Glass's 14-year-old daughter had created a model of the way social distancing might slow the spread of the flu. Glass built on it to create a simulation "proving" lockdowns could reduce an influenza epidemic in a hypothetical town of 10,000 people by 90 percent. "Dr. Mecher received the results at his office in Washington and was amazed," the Times wrote.

Robert and Laura Glass ultimately became the first two authors on a paper published in *Emerging Infectious Diseases,* a Centers for Disease Control journal, about the simulation. Inevitably, it contained a shout-out to Neil Ferguson. And sure enough, it showed the "mitigation strategies" worked.

In the retelling of this heroic lockdowns-for-all story by the Times, the conclusions of the paper took the CDC by storm. "In February 2007, the C.D.C. made their approach – bureaucratically called Non-Pharmaceutical Interventions, or NPIs – official U.S. policy."

The Albuquerque Journal told a similar tale about its hometown heroine in a May article:

> [Laura Glass's] work motivated research that resulted in the social distancing and self-isolation policies now being

used to curtail the spread of COVID-19.

"The inspiration, the sparks came from my daughter," said Robert J. Glass, a retired Sandia National Laboratories senior scientist. Glass was among those who built on Laura Glass's project to develop the vital strategies that are employed today.

(https://www.abqjournal.com/1450579/social-distancing-born-in-abq-teens-science-project.html)

The reality was different.

The 2007 CDC paper ran 108 pages and included descriptions of many possible ways to reduce transmission, from "voluntary isolation of ill adults" to "reducing density in public transit." (https://stacks.cdc.gov/view/cdc/11425)

Crucially, it also contained a "Pandemic Severity Index" that included five categories. On the low end, Category 1 represented a normal seasonal flu season, which still might kill up to 90,000 Americans. On the high end, a Category 5 pandemic, like the Spanish flu, would kill at least 1.8 million Americans.

Based on the CDC's scale, Sars-Cov-2 almost certainly should be classified as Category 2 epidemic, meaning it will cause between 90,000 and 450,000 deaths. For Category 2 or 3 epidemics, the CDC merely said governments should *consider* school closures of less than four weeks, along with moderate efforts to reduce contacts among adults, such as encouraging telecommuting.

The prospect of closing all retail stores or offices *is not even mentioned in the paper* – not even during a Category 5 epidemic killing millions of people. (The CDC's 2017 guidance, which superseded the 2007 paper, is less detailed but follows similar broad outlines. Crucially, the updated guidance lacked the "Pandemic Severity Index," ultimately giving public health officials and politicians more leeway to impose extraordinary measures.)

Yet the Times glossed over these distinctions in its article. It wrote instead "the (Bush) administration ultimately sided with the proponents of social distancing and shutdowns" and claimed the coronavirus response came directly from the original CDC report. "Then the coronavirus came, and the plan was put to work across the country for the first time."

Even as the CDC was putting its 2007 plan together, many scientists and physicians with expertise in treating pandemics worried about the weakness of real-world evidence for lockdowns and other interventions – and a potential overreliance on computer modeling.

Among the most vocal critics of lockdowns was Dr. Donald Henderson. Henderson, a recipient of the Presidential Medal of Freedom, led the successful effort to eradicate smallpox. In December 2006, Henderson and three others wrote an 11-page paper called "Disease Mitigation Measures in the Control of Pandemic Influenza." After outlining potential lockdown measures, they wrote, "We must ask whether any or all of the proposed measures are epidemiologically sound... [and] consider possible secondary social and economic impacts."

(https://www.liebertpub.com/doi/10.1089/bsp.2006.4.366?url ver=Z39.88-

Efforts in past epidemics to slow – much less stop – the spread
of the flu had largely failed, the authors wrote. They attacked
quarantines, travel bans, and school closings of more than two
weeks as likely counterproductive. They did not even mention
full lockdowns, presumably because they viewed those as so
unlikely. Near the end of the paper, they made a heartfelt plea:

> Experience has shown that
> communities faced with
> epidemics or other adverse
> events respond best and with
> the least anxiety **when the
> normal social functioning of
> the community is least
> disrupted.** [Emphasis added.]

Henderson and his co-authors were not alone in their concerns.

In 2006, the Institute of Medicine – a federally chartered non-
partisan group that offers advice on tough health questions –
held a conference to discuss flu outbreaks. Ultimately, the
institute produced a 47-page report on "modeling community
containment for pandemic influenza."

(https://www.nap.edu/catalog/11800/modeling-community-
containment-for-pandemic-influenza-a-letter-report)

The report repeatedly discussed the limitations of the research
on how epidemics spread. "A major limitation of the models is
the uncertainty in many of the assumptions," the report's
authors wrote. "There is little evidence to support many of the
key parameters."

At best, "models should be viewed as aids to decision-making, rather than substitutes for decision-making," the report warned. Unfortunately, "there is a real risk that in the midst of a crisis, there will be pressure for government to employ public health interventions, even in the absence of proven benefits."

These fears have proven prescient. And public health experts themselves were not only not immune to the panic, in many cases they seemed to lead it. Among Donald Henderson's co-authors on the 2006 paper was Dr. Thomas Inglesby, an infectious disease specialist and director of the Center for Health Security at Johns Hopkins University.

Inglesby didn't seem to change his views on lockdowns much over the next 14 years. On January 23, 2020, even as the coronavirus broke out in Hubei province, he tweeted his fear that "large scale quarantine for nCoV [the novel coronavirus] will be ineffective and could have big negative consequences." (https://twitter.com/t_inglesby/status/1220335490374742017)

Then, suddenly, he made a 180-degree turn. By April 6, he told Scientific American that the newly imposed lockdowns in the United States should not be lifted without "declines in new cases, widespread testing... and the use of nonmedical masks by the public." (https://www.scientificamerican.com/article/when-can-we-lift-the-coronavirus-pandemic-restrictions-not-before-taking-these-steps/)

I emailed and tweeted at Inglesby to ask if he saw any contradiction between the 2006 paper and his current stance, and if so how he explained the change in his views.

He did not respond.

But Inglesby was not alone in his sudden change of heart. As *The New York Times* reported in an April article about the British response to the coronavirus, top British scientists – including Neil Ferguson and the government's chief scientific advisor, Sir Patrick Vallance – had believed the United Kingdom would not need a lockdown. "Then, confronted with new numbers that projected hospitals would be overwhelmed with patients and that the death toll would skyrocket, they pivoted to a suppression strategy."
(https://www.nytimes.com/2020/04/23/world/europe/uk-coronavirus-sage-secret.html)

The early March reports of overwhelmed hospitals in northern Italy – and Italy's aggressive response – no doubt played a role. On March 9, Italy began a hard national lockdown, becoming the first country to close its entire territory. All non-essential travel was banned. Stores and government offices were shut. Police began checking more than 100,000 people a day, and thousands were fined.
(https://www.theguardian.com/world/2020/mar/18/italy-charges-more-than-40000-people-violating-lockdown-coronavirus)

Lost in the panic was the fact that Italy has had several recent severe flu epidemics. In both the 2014-15 and 2016-17 flu seasons, so-called influenza-like-illnesses killed more than 40,000 Italians – the equivalent of nearly a quarter-million Americans. Northern Italy appears to be particularly susceptible to respiratory viruses because it has a very elderly population and high levels of air pollution.
(https://www.sciencedirect.com/science/article/pii/S0269749120320601?via%3Dihub)

As the epidemic accelerated across Europe, Spain became the next major country to announce a lockdown, on Friday March 13. At that point, Imperial College still had not yet publicly released its paper projecting millions of deaths. But it had already been shown to politicians and policymakers in the United States and Europe.

"An Imperial College coronavirus model has had a profound impact on public policy since its results were shared with British and American officials **last week** [emphasis added]," the Financial Times reported on March 19. Ferguson had presented an estimate of 500,000 British deaths to a semi-secret British government scientific committee as early as February 27.

(https://www.ft.com/content/16764a22-69ca-11ea-a3c9-1fe6fedcca75)

(https://www.theguardian.com/world/2020/may/29/sage-minutes-reveal-how-uk-advisers-reacted-to-coronavirus-crisis)

The apparent success of the Chinese lockdown in quelling the epidemic in Hubei province may also have encouraged governments to consider stronger steps, although serious questions have been raised about the accuracy of the hospitalization and fatality data from China.

Journalists and historians will be sorting through the March panic for years. Only when governments fully declassify meeting notes and emails will we gain a more complete picture of what happened.

But the most likely explanation is the simplest. Faced with a risk of hundreds of thousands or millions of deaths, the public health experts who for decades had counseled patience and caution flinched. They found they could not live with acknowledging how little control they or any of us had over the spread of an easily transmissible respiratory virus. They had to do *something* – even if they had been warning for decades that what they were about to do would not work and might have terrible secondary consequences.

So lockdowns spread country to country and state to state. Even at the time, it was not clear whether the measures were intended to "flatten the curve" – to slow the spread temporarily and give hospitals a chance to get ready for a spike in cases – or to suppress the epidemic forever. No matter. The media cheered. Politicians vowed not to impose lockdowns, then changed their minds in days.

No one reversed course faster or harder than New York governor Andrew Cuomo. On Thursday, March 19, he promised that he would not impose a quarantine on his state:

> New York, and New York City in particular, will not be quarantined or force people to stay "locked up" in their homes or shelter in place. "None of that is going to happen," he said.

(https://www.nbcnews.com/health/health-news/live-blog/2020-03-19-coronavirus-news-n1163556/ncrd1163936)

The next day, Cuomo imposed a lockdown. (https://www.nydailynews.com/coronavirus/ny-coronavirus-cuomo-20200320-qrsrtcp3grfyvj5llf47cj6xoa-story.html) As he put it: "When I talk about the most drastic action we can take, this is the most drastic action we can take."

He was right.

Which didn't mean it would work.

4

Lockdowns, now

Too late.

We'd locked down too late.

As stores and offices and schools shut, as the United States braced for a surge, the fear in the media and from politicians was palpable; *the lockdowns hadn't come in time.* In New York City, the number of newly hospitalized patients with coronavirus more than tripled from 185 on March 15 to 665 on March 20. Everyone expected many more hospitalizations and deaths were coming, in New York and everywhere else. The only question was how many.

Why?

Because hospitalizations lag infections, and deaths lag hospitalizations.

Following infection with Sars-Cov-2, the average time to develop symptoms like fever or cough is five days. (https://www.ncbi.nlm.nih.gov/pmc/articles/PMC7081172/) Most people then recover relatively fast. But some get sicker. Within five to eight days, they need hospitalization. For an unlucky few, intensive care follows a day or two after, then intubation and death. In all, in the tiny fraction of cases when the novel coronavirus kills, death comes at roughly 18 days after symptoms begin and 23 days after infection. (https://www.thelancet.com/journals/laninf/article/PIIS1473-3099(20)30243-7/fulltext)

As the Atlanta Journal-Constitution explains, "epidemiologists agree that today's counts are a snapshot of what the virus did roughly two weeks ago. It can take a week or more for a person to become infected, show symptoms, get tested, and have their results reported."

(https://www.ajc.com/news/coronavirus-georgia-covid-dashboard/jvoLBozRtBSVSNQDDAuZxH/)

In other words, the people hospitalized in New York on March 20 had likely gotten sick before March 10. And they were the tip of the iceberg. The city hadn't closed schools until Monday, March 16. Offices and stores remained open during that week. But people who were infected on the 20th wouldn't show up at hospitals until the end of the month.

No one knew just how quickly infections had increased between March 10th and 20th, but the potential numbers were terrifying. Hospitalizations had risen 3.6-fold in five days. If they increased again at that rate over the next 10, the city would have almost 9,000 patients *a day* by March 30 before the lockdowns finally kicked in.

Thus Cuomo projected that coronavirus patients would soon overrun every medical center in New York. On Tuesday, March 24, he projected New York would need 140,000 hospital beds and 40,000 ventilators for them within two to three weeks – an unfathomable catastrophe.
(https://www.cnbc.com/2020/03/24/gov-cuomo-says-new-york-needs-ventilators-now-help-from-gm-ford-does-us-no-good.html).

These doomsday projections proved far off. But Cuomo wasn't making them on his own. The hospital center Weill Cornell Medicine, the consulting firm McKinsey & Company, and the CDC were all advising him. And on March 26, the Institute for

Health Metrics and Evaluation at the University of Washington released its own forecasts for all 50 states.

The IHME works closely with the Gates Foundation, which gave it $279 million in a 10-year-grant in 2017. Its mission statement says it "provides rigorous measurement and analysis of the world's most prevalent and costly health problems." Its model purported to forecast deaths, hospitalizations, and ventilator needs for every state and many countries.

IHME's forecasts predicted a terrifying future, with a sharp and unstoppable rise in cases. Within three weeks, the United States would need nearly 250,000 hospital beds for coronavirus patients, as well as more than 30,000 intensive care beds – far more than were available in many states.

Crucially, IHME released its model *after* most states had begun lockdowns, and the model assumed the shutdowns would continue until the epidemic was over. In fact, IHME assumed that even states which had not yet locked down would do so:

> [The forecasts are] predicated on the enactment of social distancing measures in all states that have not done so already within the next week and maintenance of these measures throughout the epidemic.

(http://www.healthdata.org/research-article/forecasting-covid-19-impact-hospital-bed-days-icu-days-ventilator-days-and-deaths)

Along with the rapid peak, the model assumed a quick plunge in hospitalizations after lockdowns took hold. By early May, hospitalizations nationally would fall under 100,000, and by late May below 30,000, it said.

(http://www.healthdata.org/sites/default/files/files/research_a
rticles/2020/COVID-forecasting-03252020_4.pdf)

This forecast only made sense if *lockdowns worked to reduce
transmission, quickly and certainly.* Like the Imperial College
model, the IHME model assumed the epidemic would spread
uncontrolled before hard lockdowns but rapidly shrink
thereafter, as R – the transmission rate – fell below 1.

Overnight, the IHME model became the crucial forecasting tool
for state and federal governments. On April 8, the Washington
Post called it "America's Most Influential Coronavirus Model."
(Any criticism came mostly from epidemiologists who believed
its forecasts were too rosy.)

(https://www.washingtonpost.com/health/2020/04/06/americ
as-most-influential-coronavirus-model-just-revised-its-
estimates-downward-not-every-model-agrees/)

In the 10 days after the institute released the model, it
repeatedly revised upwards its forecasts for hospitalizations and
ventilator use. For example, on April 5, the revised IHME model
projected that New York would need 69,000 hospital beds and
almost 10,000 ventilators *that day.*

What no one in the media or at the Institute for Health Metrics
and Evaluation seemed to care about – or even notice – was
that the model had failed completely. It was failing not just to
predict the future but accurately measure what was happening
in real time.

On April 5, New York actually had about 16,500 people in
hospitals – fewer than one-quarter the number **the model
claimed were hospitalized that day**. Of those, about 4,000
patients, not 10,000, were on ventilators.

Why did the IHME model fail just days after it was released? Why did it and the other models so badly overestimate the number of patients who would be hospitalized with the coronavirus?

The institute and its director, Dr. Christopher Murray, did not return emails for comment.

But the simplest answer for the model's crucial initial failure is that growth in hospitalizations in New York slowed much faster than it forecast. After their 3.6-fold rise between March 15 and March 20, new admissions doubled again by March 25, to 1,323. Then their exponential growth abruptly ended.

Over the next two weeks, they stayed in the range of 1,300 to 1,700 a day, before beginning a rapid decline. (Overall hospitalizations actually peaked earlier and declined faster, as patients began to be discharged fairly quickly.)

In most other states, hospitalizations in late March never really accelerated. The model proved just as inaccurate everywhere else, though off a lower base.

An aside: no one can blame the failure of the models on lack of compliance with the lockdowns. All over the world, most people accepted the measures as unfortunate but necessary. Businesses, offices, and schools closed. Air travel nearly vanished. Even as the lockdowns stretched deep into April, most Americans and Europeans stayed home without much complaint.

A combination of fear, public pressure, and a genuine desire to support frontline health-care workers seems to have driven obedience. Heavy media and corporate propaganda helped. Endless television ads aimed to convince people to "come together by staying apart." (By mid-April, an advertising copywriter named Samantha Geloso had created a hilarious spoof, but that didn't stop the ads. https://adage.com/creativity/work/montage-takes-piss-out-pandemic-montages/2250301)

By mid-April, some Americans – mostly conservatives – had begun to demand an end to the lockdowns. But their protests made little difference. Media outlets like CNN and the Times, which fully supported the lockdowns, treated the protests as fringe events. They never gained enough momentum to matter. The governors who locked down their states the hardest saw the *biggest* jumps in their approval ratings.

Data from Apple on mobility shows how effective the lockdowns were. Across the United States, driving dropped 25 percent in the week before March 20, then fell another 50 percent before bottoming out on Sunday, April 12. Mass transit use bottomed the same day, down 80 percent from normal levels. (https://www.apple.com/covid19/mobility) Overall, American mobility dropped almost two-thirds from early March to mid-April before slowly recovering.

That figure was less than lockdown champions such as Italy – where the drop was more than 80 percent and lasted even longer – or the United Kingdom. But it was comparable to countries like Germany and higher than many people might have predicted before the lockdowns began.

Further, the national data don't catch the impact of the lockdowns in hard-hit areas. In New York City, driving bottomed out at 30 percent of normal, mass transit use at barely 10 percent. Even those figures underestimate the way the city *felt*. Hundreds of thousands of people fled New York in March and

April. Aside from police officers, medical staff, and other essential workers, almost no one went outside. The empty streets and shuttered stores were eerie, as I saw for myself on repeated trips.

No, the failure or success of lockdowns can't be blamed on lack of compliance.

What, then? The IHME model and its cousins badly overestimated hospitalizations. But their failures didn't end with that error. They were wrong *both on the way up and the way down.* The models predicted a short peak and rapid decline, but hospitals emptied slowly.

And although the models overestimated hospitalizations, they *underestimated* the number and timing of deaths. In its various revisions, IHME predicted between 60,000 and 90,000 American deaths by August, with deaths falling sharply after a mid-April peak. The United States currently has about 150,000 reported deaths, and deaths both in the United States and elsewhere dropped only slowly.

In Britain, Ferguson made a similar mistake when he reduced his estimate of deaths from 500,000 to 25,000 on March 25. Britain has now had 46,000 deaths.

The simulations designed by the world's top epidemiologists failed in every way.

Why?

The most likely answer has everything to do with lockdowns. *The failure of the models cannot be separated from the failure of lockdowns.* Neil Ferguson and the epidemiologists designing the models believed that lockdowns worked, that they were the only way to make the epidemic manageable.

But they misunderstood the fact that lockdowns failed utterly to protect the people most at risk.

The worst coronavirus outbreaks have followed the same pattern everywhere – whether Wuhan in January, northern Italy in early March, or New York and London a few days later. In a densely populated area, Sars-Cov-2 spreads quietly but quickly for days or weeks – a Chinese researcher estimated that the R might have been close to 3.9 in Wuhan in January, a rate that if unchecked means 1 infection would become more than 3,000 in a month. (https://docs.google.com/presentation/d/1-rvZsOzsXF_0Tw8TNsBxKH4V1LQQXq7Az9kDfCgZDfE/edit#slide=id.p32)

The illness then jumps into public view as conventional and social media fill with doomsday predictions. And as a lockdown is considered, even if it is initially rejected, the panic rises still further. Although people may begin to travel less and voluntarily socially distance during this period, emergency room visits and 911 calls soar, driven both by fear and real viral spread.

In New York, emergency room visits for respiratory and flu-like symptoms rose from about 1,700 a day at the beginning of March to more than 4,000 by the middle of the month. Some people already had coronavirus or the flu. Others were simply afraid. For them, emergency rooms were an ideal ground to pick up or trade the virus. They also increase the risk of passing the virus to the physicians and medical staff who treat them – who in turn can spread it to patients who are already hospitalized.

This pattern rapidly became clear to front-line doctors. As early as March 21, a group of physicians in northern Italy warned in a New England Journal of Medicine article:

> We are learning that hospitals might be the main Covid-19

carriers, as they are rapidly populated by infected patients, facilitating transmission to uninfected patients. Patients are transported by our regional system, which also contributes to spreading the disease as its ambulances and personnel rapidly become vectors...

[Sars-Cov-2] is not particularly lethal, but it is very contagious. The more medicalized and centralized the society, the more widespread the virus.

(https://catalyst.nejm.org/doi/full/10.1056/CAT.20.0080?fbclid=IwAR0wa6jzq-t_YYlZlYQtWiVmphT8pjyGBCndLhJGSN34dBaeZJoGP0sfneo)

In other words, panic itself drives vulnerable people to hospitals and thus increases transmission among them. And nothing causes panic to spike faster than the serious consideration of lockdowns.

At the same time, lockdowns force people to stay inside. (Obviously. That's the *point* of lockdowns.)

Unfortunately, coronavirus spreads most efficiently inside, especially in households living in poorly ventilated apartments or small houses, their windows closed against winter cold or summer heat. On March 30, Dr. Mike Ryan, the Irish surgeon who leads the World Health Organization's COVID containment and treatment program, warned at a WHO press conference:

At the moment, in most parts of the world, due to lockdown, most of the transmission that's actually happening in many countries now is happening in the household at family level. In some senses, transmission has been taken off the streets and pushed back into family units.

(https://www.youtube.com/watch?v=2v3vlw14NbM&feature=youtu.be&t=2996, at approximately 50:00.)

[Ryan's solution to this problem was to propose forcibly isolating infected patients and quarantining their family members, but that's a story for another day, and a later section of Unreported Truths.]

All over the world, researchers and government agencies have reached the same conclusion. On April 7, Chinese researchers published a paper that looked at 318 outbreaks with 1,245 Sars-Cov-2 infections. They found that 80 percent took place in homes or apartments. Another 34 percent occurred on public transportation (some outbreaks occurred in more than one place, or could not be placed at a single venue). All other venues, including stores and restaurants, accounted for less than 20 percent of infections combined.

"Sharing indoor space is a major SARS-CoV-2 infection risk," the researchers wrote.

(https://www.medrxiv.org/content/10.1101/2020.04.04.20053058v1)

Similarly, in examining a week of cases from June 28 through July 4, the Health Ministry of Quebec reported fewer than 15 percent could be traced to workplaces, stores, or bars and restaurants. 35 percent were intra-familial. Another 25 percent were of health care workers, patients, or prison inmates, and a similar number could not be traced. Particularly striking about the Quebec figures is that they occurred after the province's lockdown had ended.

(https://www.cbc.ca/news/canada/montreal/covid-19-quebec-why-are-cases-increasing-1.5658082)

In other words, in the short run, increasing the amount of time family members spend with each other may drive up transmission.

Even worse, the people most vulnerable to that intra-familial transmission of coronavirus – the extremely elderly and people with severe health problems – rarely work and are the *least* likely to spend time outside. They are naturally somewhat protected, until lockdowns confine them with family members who have been infected elsewhere and bring the virus home.

Worst of all, broad lockdowns do not appear to make much difference to the spread of the virus in nursing homes. Long-term care facilities are uniquely vulnerable to the coronavirus because their patients are both medically fragile and live close together. Fewer than 0.5 percent of Americans live in nursing homes – fewer than 1 in 200 people. But in both the United States and Europe, nursing home residents have accounted for 40 to 50 percent of all Covid deaths, well over 100,000 in all. (https://www.theguardian.com/world/2020/may/16/across-the-world-figures-reveal-horrific-covid-19-toll-of-care-home-deaths)

Even during lockdowns, nursing homes and other "congregate care" facilities cannot close. How to protect them, then? Measures such as frequently testing staff members and patients, ensuring the homes have adequate cleaning equipment, and quickly hospitalizing infected residents may help contain outbreaks.

But the effort required to promote and manage lockdowns can distract governments from the crisis in nursing homes. In northern Italy, as a strict lockdowns dragged on, "nursing homes were in many ways left to fend for themselves," an Associated Press article reported on April 26. (https://www.whsv.com/content/news/Perfect-storm-Lombardys-virus-disaster-is-lesson-for-world-569961341.html) The panic that lockdowns foment may even play a role in causing staff to flee and leaving residents without care, as happened in Spain. (https://www.npr.org/sections/coronavirus-live-updates/2020/03/24/820711855/spanish-military-finds-dead-bodies-and-seniors-completely-abandoned-in-care-home)

The fact that lockdowns do little to help nursing homes may be one reason that deaths go on so long after they begin – contrary to the forecasts from IHME and others. The United Kingdom, which has had more deaths per-capita than any other big country, imposed a lockdown nearly as strict as Italy's on March 23. Deaths peaked April 10 at about 1100 a day, but remained around 630 a day almost four weeks later. And more than 16,000 of the deaths occurred in nursing homes.

Six months into the epidemic, the data are clear: the overall number of people infected with Sars-Cov-2 is less relevant to the number of people who die than *which people are infected*. Only when nursing home and hospital outbreaks burn out do deaths decrease.

An April 15 paper from the Robert Koch Institute, Germany's equivalent of the Centers for Disease Control, offers a slightly different perspective on the issue.

In the paper, researchers there tracked the number of infections in Germany for more than two months. They found that the spread of the virus peaked at the beginning of March. At that point each newly person infected 3 others – an R of 3, showing just how contagious Sars-Cov-2 can naturally be. Over the next three weeks the transmission rate fell to around 1.

(https://www.rki.de/DE/Content/Infekt/EpidBull/Archiv/2020/Ausgaben/17_20_SARS-CoV2_vorab.pdf?__blob=publicationFile)

Yet Germany imposed a hard lockdown *late* – on March 23, two weeks after Italy's.

What happened? Southern Germany is not even 200 miles from the northern Italian border. Reports about the burgeoning outbreak in Italy apparently prompted Germans to take their own voluntary social distancing measures and reduce the spread of the virus – *before* the damaging panic that comes with the consideration and imposition of a lockdown.

The lockdown itself reduced the transmission marginally more, to 0.9. But it did little to protect vulnerable populations, the report warned. "After March 18 the virus spreads more to older people and we are also increasingly seeing outbreaks in nursing homes and hospitals."

Still, Germany made containing outbreaks in nursing homes a priority. And it wound up with a fraction of the nursing home deaths – or overall deaths – in Britain, Italy, or Spain.

(https://www.theguardian.com/world/2020/jun/28/covid-19-risk-of-death-in-uk-care-homes-13-times-higher-than-in-germany)

Yet more evidence that lockdowns were ineffective came after American states and European countries lifted them. Denmark was the first European country to end its lockdowns, reopening schools in April and stores by early May. More than a month later, on June 10, the Danish national health authority reported that "there is no sign yet of noticeable changes." Switzerland and other European countries noted similar trends.

(https://www.reuters.com/article/us-health-coronavirus-denmark/denmark-sees-no-rise-in-covid-19-cases-after-further-easing-of-lockdown-idUSKBN23H1DU)

In the United States, southern states began lifting lockdowns as early as April 24, led by Georgia. The decision led to predictable media hysteria. The Atlantic magazine infamously called the decision "Georgia's Experiment In Human Sacrifice."

Yet the United States saw no spike in coronavirus cases in May or early June. On May 20, Marko Kolanovic, a senior strategist at J.P. Morgan (like Neil Ferguson, a physicist by training), analyzed reopening and transmission data. He concluded that the virus had actually spread more slowly in the United States after lockdowns ended.

Then, in June, cases began to rise in a broad stretch of states from California to Florida. Hospitalizations followed. In Arizona, the first state to see a major spike, hospitalizations more than tripled from roughly 1,000 on June 1 to 3,500 on July 13. In Texas, the spike began later but was even sharper, from 2,000 on June 11 to almost 11,000 on July 22. Florida saw a similar trend, with hospitalizations rising from roughly 2,000 to almost 9,000.

Deaths also surged in all three states, though with a predictable lag. (Death reporting is tricky not just because the criteria for counting deaths as Covid-related are extremely loose but because some deaths are reported almost immediately while others are not counted for weeks or even months.) By any count, though, hospitalizations and especially deaths have occurred at a far lower level than the Northeast in March.

Several different and plausible explanations for the Sunbelt spike have been offered – including the heavy use of air conditioning, young people deciding not to protect themselves because they now know they are at low risk, and possibly even some importation of cases from Mexico. That confused reality has not stopped media outlets from insisting that the end of lockdowns must have been responsible for the rise in infections – even though the rise began between five and eight weeks after the lockdowns ended.

Even more importantly, the media has largely failed to report that the *Sunbelt spike in hospitalizations is over.* Arizona, Florida, and Texas have all seen big drops in hospitalizations in late July. The drop is most stunning in Arizona, where cases peaked first. Between July 13 and August 3, hospitalizations fell to just over 2,000 – a drop of almost 50 percent. In Texas, hospitalized Covid patients fell from their July 22 peak to under 9,000 by August 3, a drop of almost 20 percent. In all three states, hospitals were stressed, but none faced overrun and the overall quality of care either Covid or other patients received appeared unaffected.

Further, in all three states, the drop in hospitalizations came *despite the fact the states did not reimpose widespread lockdowns,* though they did take minor steps to slow the spread of the virus and reduce the strain on hospitals. Arizona closed gyms and bars, for example, while Florida closed bars and Texas postponed elective surgeries. (Neither Arizona nor Florida mandated masks, either, although Texas required them in most counties.)

About 180 years ago, a British epidemiologist and statistician named William Farr examined data from smallpox and other epidemics and concluded that in viral epidemics, deaths tend *to both rise and fall* in a roughly symmetrical pattern that looks like a bell curve – a long tail followed by a quick rise followed by a rounded peak, with a sharp drop and a long tail on the other side.

What's so striking about Farr's observation is that the type of virus and its lethality and transmissibility don't seem to matter as much as our (voluntary) human response to the virus – and the gradual growth in the number of people who have been infected by and recovered from the virus and can no longer pass it on. Further, Farr noted that epidemics generally strike the most vulnerable first and hardest: "The most mortal die out." As a result, early estimates of mortality may be hugely overstated.

(https://www.sciencedirect.com/science/article/pii/S2468042718300101)

(https://www.cebm.net/covid-19/covid-19-william-farrs-way-out-of-the-pandemic/#:~:text=Farr%20showed%20that%20epidemics%20rise,pattern%20on%20the%20downward%20slope.)

The shape of the hospitalization curves in Arizona couldn't fit Farr's law better – a bell curve with a rounded peak and a sharp drop. Lockdown or not, a simple theory did a far better job of predicting the course of the epidemic there than powerful computer simulations.

Any worldwide review of lockdowns must touch on three other countries: Sweden, New Zealand, and Japan.

Sweden has attracted a huge amount of attention as the only major Western European country to refuse to lockdown. At first glance, Sweden appears to provide evidence for both pro- and anti-lockdown views. Per-capita death coronavirus rates there are lower than Britain or Italy, though higher than Germany or the Nordic countries.

In fact, though, Sweden's high death rates were driven almost entirely by the fact that the country didn't just fail to protect nursing homes but in some cases actually discouraged physicians from offering care to the extremely elderly. In a June article headline, "Coronavirus Is Taking a High Toll on Sweden's Elderly. Families Blame the Government," *The Wall Street Journal* detailed disturbing cases in which older patients had been refused hospitalizations.
(https://www.wsj.com/articles/coronavirus-is-taking-a-high-toll-on-swedens-elderly-families-blame-the-government-11592479430)

As a result, Sweden's coronavirus deaths skew extremely elderly. Almost two-thirds of deaths occurred in people 80 or over, and almost 90 percent in people 70 or over. The Swedish government has acknowledged that its failure to protect nursing homes was a huge and preventable error.

Overall, the course of the epidemic in Sweden has essentially tracked that of countries like Italy and Spain – a big early spike, followed by a slow decline. The trend suggests lockdowns are irrelevant, and that protecting nursing homes makes far more difference.

On the other hand, the most impressive country-level evidence in favor of lockdowns comes from New Zealand, which locked down very hard and very early, and now appears to have largely eliminated the coronavirus on its territory. But – like

Newfoundland, a Canadian province that took similar steps — New Zealand is an exceptional case, a lightly populated and isolated island that plays a minor role in global commerce and can easily shut its borders.

Those states may be the *only* ones with a realistic chance of using lockdowns to control the coronavirus, as long as they are willing to enforce long-term border quarantines and aggressively track any positive case; whether the dangers of the virus justify such steps is a question more political than scientific. And even in those areas, any relaxation of the rules may lead to a quick spike in cases, as Hawaii — which until recently appeared to have controlled the virus effectively — is now learning.

If New Zealand offers the strongest case for lockdowns, Japan offers the opposite. Japan should have been ground zero for the epidemic. It has one of the world's oldest populations, one of its largest cities, heavy reliance on mass transit, and close air links to China. Its poor performance quarantining the ill-fated *Diamond Princess* cruise ship in February suggested its authorities lacked basic infection control awareness. "Health officials and even some medical professionals worked on board without full protective gear," the Times reported on Feb. 22. (https://www.nytimes.com/2020/02/22/world/asia/coronavirus -japan-cruise-ship.html)

And Japan never imposed a full national lockdown, instead in April imposing only a partial "state of emergency" that lasted only a few weeks and consisted of largely voluntary restrictions. As Bloomberg News wrote in May:

> No restrictions were placed on residents' movements, and businesses from restaurants to hairdressers stayed open. No

high-tech apps that tracked people's movements were deployed. The country doesn't have a center for disease control. And even as nations were exhorted to "test, test, test," Japan has tested just 0.2% of its population -- one of the lowest rates among developed countries.

Yet Japan has had an almost bizarrely easy time with Sars-Cov-2. It has reported about 250 cases per million people, even fewer than New Zealand, and 8 deaths per million – about 1 percent of Britain's rate.

Why? No one really knows. Many Japanese wear masks in public, especially if they have fever or cough, although masking is far from universal. Authorities also discouraged people from gathering in crowds, in closed spaces like bars, and talking closely – the "three Cs" strategy.

(https://www.sciencemag.org/news/2020/05/japan-ends-its-covid-19-state-emergency?utm_campaign=news_daily_2020-05-26&et_rid=687438071&et_cid=3340566)

If those explanations seem unsatisfying, it's because they are. But we can be sure lockdowns are *not* the reason for Japan's success. Yet American public health experts have for the most part simply *ignored* Japan and simply continued to snipe at Sweden, rather than doing the hard work of grappling with their policy choices and apparent successes.

One last point: scientific journals have recently published several papers purporting to show that lockdowns saved hundreds of thousands or even millions of lives. Not to put too fine a point on it, these papers are junk – mathematical models created in some cases by the very same epidemiologists whose forecasts four months ago proved entirely wrong. And these models are even more useless, because they aren't even trying to predict the future but instead describing an alternative past that didn't take place and thus cannot be proven true or false.

For example, in June, Imperial College researchers (yes, again) put out a paper claiming that lockdowns might have saved *millions* of lives in Europe. Beyond the fact that the researchers used an estimate for the virus's risk of death far higher than the current best estimates, they looked at 10 European countries. They found that lockdowns, however and whenever they were exposed, had worked in all 10.

(https://www.nature.com/articles/s41586-020-2405-7)

But they included Sweden as a lockdown country.

Which unintentionally made the point exactly the opposite of the one they intended. After all, if Sweden had the same results as everywhere else, how can anyone think lockdowns made a difference?

Considered as whole, the evidence – at best – suggests hard lockdowns *may* eventually slow the general spread of the coronavirus. After all, following months of lockdowns, the epidemic in Italy, Spain, and New York did burn out.

Even that case is not proven, as Sweden shows. With or without lockdowns, some hard-hit countries and regions may eventually reach "herd immunity." Essentially, herd immunity occurs when so many people have already been infected and recovered and developed antibodies that the virus can no longer move freely through the population.

But the debate over what percentage of the population must be infected before herd immunity is reached is both highly technical and subject to many of the modeling uncertainties that have proven so damaging already. So it's best left for later.

What lockdown proponents seem to forget is a general gradual slowdown makes little difference, especially for a virus whose risks are as skewed to the elderly and sick as Sars-Cov-2. What matters is breaking spikes that can cause hospital overrun, while protecting the vulnerable. General lockdowns do neither. And because of the fear they provoke and the leadership attention they require to promote and implement, they are a distraction from focusing on those in need of protection at the worst possible time.

Even the WHO seems to have recognized the futility of lockdowns. In a recent interview with the British newspaper The Telegraph, Dr. Maria Van Kerkhove, a leader of the organization's coronavirus response team, discouraged countries from reimposing lockdowns. They are a "blunt, sheer force instrument" with severe social and economic consequences, she said.

(https://www.telegraph.co.uk/global-health/science-and-disease/exclusive-top-disease-detective-warns-against-return-national/)

Some European leaders have publicly admitted lockdowns were a mistake. In July, Jean Castex, the French prime minister, said the country would never again "impose a lockdown like the one did last March, because we've learned… that the economic and human consequences from a total lockdown are disastrous."

(https://www.france24.com/en/20200708-france-rules-out-total-lockdown-in-case-of-covid-19-surge)

Yes, the economic and human consequences. I thought I'd write a lot about those in this section, but I haven't bothered, because they are so self-evident. More than 50 million Americans have filed for unemployment; the United States economy shrank by 1/3 in the second quarter on an annualized basis, the sharpest drop ever recorded.

The damage goes far beyond bank accounts. Since March, drug overdose deaths have spiked from New Jersey to British Columbia; murders have soared in many big American cities. (We don't know exactly how much, because although we obsessively count coronavirus deaths in real-time, we pay far less attention to other causes of death.) Millions of "elective" surgeries have been postponed worldwide, leading to untold misery for patients suffering from chronic pain, failing joints, and other ailments, and even death in the cases of people needing heart surgery or cancer care.

(https://www.dailymail.co.uk/news/article-8396253/UK-patients-face-TWO-YEAR-wait-elective-surgery-NHS-backlog-set-hit-650-000.html)

(https://nowtoronto.com/news/april-28-coronavirus-updates-toronto-news)

Hundreds of millions of children worldwide have been denied the chance to learn and play at school. Anxiety and depression are soaring; on social media people proudly and publicly self-report that they have not gone outside for months.
(https://www.washingtonpost.com/health/2020/05/04/mental-health-coronavirus/)

The lockdowns have punished all of us (except technology and social media companies, which are reporting record profits) enormously. Which might not matter if we had compelling evidence they worked.

Only we don't.

So the calls by some members of Team Apocalypse for *renewed* lockdowns – even *harder* lockdowns, in fact, as if we didn't do enough damage in the spring – might sound like a joke. Especially since hospitals even in the hardest-hit Sunbelt states are beginning to empty. But they're not a joke. They're serious – as the decision on Aug. 2 by the Australian province of Victoria to impose a new and draconian lockdown on Melbourne, a city with 5 million people, shows.

Lockdowns have failed as badly as the experts warned us they would, for precisely the reasons those experts spent their careers predicting. But the hysterics have learned nothing from the last four months.

Experience has shown that communities faced with epidemics or other adverse events respond best and with the least anxiety when the normal social functioning of the community is least disrupted.

Those words are as true now as they were in 2006. We have forgotten them once already this year.

We can't afford to make that mistake again.

UNREPORTED TRUTHS ABOUT COVID-19 AND LOCKDOWNS:

PART 3:

Masks

(Published November 24, 2020)

5

I wish masks worked.

I wish masks worked. If they did they'd be a cheap, easy way to slow the spread of Sars-Cov-2.

I wish masks worked. The idea they protect not just their wearers but also the people around them seems wonderfully selfless.

I wish masks worked. Americans are spending billions of dollars on them and they can cause acne and frighten small children and people with disabilities. Wearing them for no reason seems perverse.

I wish masks worked. Most Americans now wear them. Telling people they have been conned doesn't make them happy.

I wish masks worked. They have become *the* flashpoint in the political battles around Sars-Cov-2. Anyone who opposes wearing masks, much less making everyone wear them, draws scorn from the media and scientific establishment. *Bet you think the virus is fake, too. People are dying!*

I wish masks worked. We have so many other battles to fight around coronavirus: lockdowns, school closings, travel restrictions, and other government intrusions into our lives. Masks seem at first like one that isn't worth the trouble. *Wear a mask,* the advocates insist. *Stop arguing, just wear it. It's nothing.*

I wish masks worked.

But they don't.

Not the ordinary cloth and surgical masks that nearly everybody wears, anyway. Despite everything the media and public health experts have told you, *they don't work.*

More accurately, we have no real evidence they do – and plenty of evidence they don't.

Welcome to Part 3 of Unreported Truths: masks. As protection, masks are largely useless, and mask mandates even more so. But as a symbol that the coronavirus is a serious danger requiring us to give up our rights, they are incredibly effective.

A lot has happened since the last installment came out in August. President Trump was infected with Sars-Cov-2 and recovered. A new outbreak raced across Europe and the United States. Several drug and biotechnology companies announced positive results for vaccines.

And Joe Biden narrowly won the presidential election, eking out a coin flip win over Donald Trump. (Whatever you think of mail-in ballots, Republicans have found no evidence of large-scale vote fraud. We should all assume Biden will take the oath of office in January.)

Elections have consequences, Barack Obama famously said. The 2020 presidential election surely will, especially for the way we respond to the coronavirus.

Biden, who was rarely photographed without a mask during the campaign, has already promised to try to make all Americans wear masks. "We can save tens of thousands of lives if everyone would just wear a mask," he said at a press conference on Nov. 9.

(https://www.nbcnews.com/politics/2020-election/biden-kicks-presidential-transition-begging-americans-wear-masks-n1247143)

Biden's official Website, "Buildbackbetter.com," calls for:

"Every American to wear a mask when they are around people outside their household.

"Every Governor to make that mandatory in their state.

"Local authorities to also make it mandatory to buttress their state orders."

Biden's proposal makes no distinction between requiring masks indoors and outdoors, or only when strangers are close together. Its language suggests Biden wants to force all of us to wear masks all the time, except when we are home with only family members around.

Biden's win also emboldened public health authorities to press masks even harder. A week after Election Day, the Centers for Disease Control issued a new advisory in which it claimed even cloth masks reduce the risk of infection in the people who wear them. The CDC wrote:

> Masks are primarily intended to reduce the emission of virus-laden droplets ("source control")... Masks also help reduce inhalation of these droplets by the wearer ("filtration for personal protection").

(https://www.cdc.gov/coronavirus/2019-ncov/more/masking-science-sars-cov2.html)

The CDC's promise that cloth and surgical masks protect the people wearing them is notable. It stands in marked contrast to what pro-mask epidemiologists have said since April. Usually, they focus on the protection masks supposedly offer to *other* people ("My mask protects you, your mask protects me.")

So why the change? The CDC decided to talk up personal protection in the hope of convincing people who aren't wearing masks to do so, according to NBC News:

> Infectious disease doctors who have urged the CDC to change the messaging around masks believe it will be a more effective public health strategy. "I'm thrilled that it's happening now," said Dr. Monica Gandhi, professor of medicine at the University of California San Francisco. "I think it helps people comply with the regulation if they think it's helping them."

(https://www.nbcnews.com/health/health-news/two-way-street-cdc-report-says-masks-protect-wearers-everyone-n1247258)

The not very well-hidden subtext here: People who are too selfish to wear masks to protect *others* might do so for their own safety.

Biden's request for *local* governments to press for mandatory mask-wearing is also notable. For the most part, states have led the push for masks, focusing on businesses rather than individuals. State health departments now make stores, restaurants, and offices require masks for entry. But local police departments have generally avoided arresting people for going maskless. The mention of "local authorities" looks to be Biden's backdoor way to change that.

Still, law enforcement is not the main driver of mask use. Public pressure is.

Ironically, in February and March, as the epidemic was taking off, the pressure came the other way. Health experts discouraged the public from using face coverings. On Feb. 29, Dr. Jerome Adams, the Surgeon General, tweeted a warning that would become infamous:

> Seriously people – STOP BUYING MASKS! They are NOT effective in preventing general public from catching #Coronavirus, but if healthcare providers can't get them to care for sick patients, it puts them and our communities at risk!

A week later, on March 8, Dr. Anthony Fauci, the director of the National Institute of Allergy and Infectious Diseases, told 60 Minutes:

> There's no reason to be walking around with a mask. When you're in the middle of an outbreak, wearing a mask might make people feel a little bit better and it might even block a droplet, but it's not providing the perfect protection that people think that it is. And, often, there are unintended consequences — people keep fiddling with the mask and they keep touching their face."

The World Health Organization also warned against wearing masks. "WHO stands by recommendation to not wear masks if you are not sick or not caring for someone who is sick," CNN reported on March 30.

On April 1, the *New England Journal of Medicine* – the leading American health-care journal – wrote:

We know that wearing a mask outside health care facilities offers little, if any, protection from infection... In many cases, the desire for widespread masking is a reflexive reaction to anxiety over the pandemic.[1]

But within days of that article, health experts reversed course and insisted people must wear masks – whether they were feeling sick or well, whether they were in hospitals or stores or even outside.

On April 22, Dr. Adams – he of "STOP BUYING MASKS" – unveiled the new mantra at a White House press conference: "You wear your mask to protect me... I wear my mask to protect you."

(https://www.whitehouse.gov/briefings-statements/remarks-president-trump-vice-president-pence-members-coronavirus-task-force-press-briefing-30/)

As states rolled back lockdowns in May and June, the advice became more strident. Masks were now the most important step to slow the epidemic. Face coverings were crucial not just for people with Covid but for those without, because even people without symptoms could spread the disease.

By June 3, the authors of the April 1 New England Journal of Medicine were claiming readers had misunderstood their original piece:

---

[1](https://twitter.com/surgeon_general/status/1233725785283932160?lang=en)

(https://www.reuters.com/article/uk-factcheck-fauci-outdated-video-masks/fact-checkoutdated-video-of-fauci-saying-theres-no-reason-to-be-walking-around-with-a-mask-idUSKBN26T2TR)

(https://www.cnn.com/2020/03/30/world/coronavirus-who-masks-recommendation-trnd/index.html)

(https://www.nejm.org/doi/full/10.1056/NEJMp2006372)

> We understand that some people are citing our Perspective article... as support for discrediting widespread masking. In truth, the intent of our article was to push for more masking, not less.

(https://www.nejm.org/doi/full/10.1056/NEJMc2020836)

Sure. The statement that masks outside hospitals offer *"little if any protection from infection"* was meant to encourage their use.

But the same media outlets which failed to ask questions about the need for lockdowns were just as credulous on the sudden 180-degree turn over masks. News organizations happily accepted the excuse by public health authorities that they had initially offered anti-mask advice only to prevent a run on masks that healthcare workers needed. In newspapers and on cable networks, pro-mask messages became the norm.

"Overnight, masks have become a symbol of social responsibility," The New York Times wrote on April 10. "If you still need convincing, here's why you now should be wearing a mask in public spaces." Two months later, the Times cheerily offered "Tips for Making Your Mask Work."

The Washington Post took slightly longer. On April 17, it called mask-wearing a "tough decision" and noted many states had originally enacted anti-mask laws to combat the Ku Klux Klan. On May 1, it warned that masks could cause painful rashes and acne for their wearers:

> Skin irritation from wearing personal protective equipment is a hazard already familiar to health-care providers working in settings where infection control is critical. Now it has also

become familiar to many people wearing masks
in public.

But by June, the Post was fully on board, explaining how "new
research supports wearing masks to control coronavirus
spread."[2]

The next step followed logically.

Having decreed masks could save people from Sars-Cov-2,
media outlets tried to embarrass anyone who refused. Not to
wear a mask was to refuse to "follow the science" – a
catchphrase repeated endlessly – and a sign of selfishness.

Newspapers and magazines published insufferably arrogant
pieces telling readers how to deal with the cretins who wouldn't
wear masks. "It can be difficult to find common ground with
someone who refuses to wear a mask for whatever reason,"
Teen Vogue wrote in July. "You might find the most resistance
from people who are ideologically opposed to wearing masks
because they believe doing so is a sign of weakness (it isn't)."

(https://www.teenvogue.com/story/how-to-talk-to-people-who-wont-wear-face-masks)

The Washington Post went a step further, warning in
September, "Some Covid-19 rule-breakers could be narcissists,
experts say. Here's how to approach them – " as if people
who'd decided to keep their faces uncovered were inherently

---

[2] https://www.nytimes.com/2020/04/10/well/live/coronavirus-face-masks-
guides-protection-personal-protective-equipment.html

https://www.nytimes.com/interactive/2020/06/25/burst/how-to-get-the-
most-out-of-your-mask.html

https://www.washingtonpost.com/health/tips-on-alleviating-face-masks-rashes-and-skin-
irritations/2020/05/01/5dd3f2ac-88b0-11ea-ac8a-fe9b8088e101_story.html

https://www.washingtonpost.com/health/2020/06/13/spate-new-
research-supports-wearing-masks-control-coronavirus-spread/

dangerous. The article even offered strategies to approach those awful narcissists. Craig Malkin, a psychologist, suggested telling them how important they were:

> "For example, [say] 'You can make the difference between life and death because we're all in this together.'"

> "The less significant they feel in all of this, the more they're going to have to pound their chests and push back against what's being expected to feel like they matter," Malkin said.

(https://www.washingtonpost.com/lifestyle/wellness/narcissism-mask-covid-psychology/2020/09/25/d3de1b32-fe9c-11ea-9ceb-061d646d9c67_story.html)

In August, a study would take this argument to the extreme. People who didn't wear masks were no longer just dumb or self-centered. They were sociopaths:

> New research from Brazil has found that people who are unconcerned with adhering to measures to prevent the spread of Covid-19 tend to display higher levels of traits associated with antisocial personality disorder, also known as sociopathy.

(https://www.news-medical.net/news/20200824/Sociopaths-less-likely-to-comply-with-COVID-mask-hygiene-and-social-distancing.aspx)

The relentless pressure has caused a sharp rise in mask wearing. In blue states like California, masks are essentially standard, even outside. People who wear masks are increasingly willing to challenge people who don't. I live in New York and try not to wear a mask outside, so I have seen the change in attitudes firsthand. Recently, a masked woman in her sixties asked me if I would step aside since she needed to walk around me and I wasn't wearing a mask. We were standing several feet apart on a hiking trail.

National surveys confirm mask wearing has risen substantially. In June, about 65 percent of Americans said they wore masks in stores all or most of the time, according to Pew Research. By August the figure had risen to 85 percent. (https://www.pewresearch.org/fact-tank/2020/08/27/more-americans-say-they-are-regularly-wearing-masks-in-stores-and-other-businesses/)

Other surveys show even more mask use.

Those percentages might slightly overstate real-world mask wearing, for the same reason polls understated Trump's support. People don't like to admit they deviate from media-promoted social norms. Still, mask wearing is clearly now the default, indoors everywhere and outdoors in most states.

Which is why it may be so surprising that the United States is now going through its third and apparently largest wave of coronavirus infections. The first and second epidemics were largely regional: the spring wave in the Northeast and Midwest, the summer outbreak in the Sunbelt. The fall outbreak seems to be everywhere. The number of reported infections – which the media calls "cases," though they are based mainly on test results and include many people with no symptoms – has reached record highs.

The number of positive tests overstates the scope of the fall epidemic because the United States now tests more than 10 million people a week, far more than it did during the spring. Further, many positive tests represent people who *had* rather than currently have Sars-Cov-2 infections. (I may address the details of the issues around PCR tests in a future booklet; they are technical but crucially important.)

Still, hospitalizations are also rising. More than 80,000 Americans are now hospitalized with the coronavirus, more than the spring or summer peaks. The growth in testing is partially driving that rise. A significant fraction of those patients have been hospitalized for other problems. They are then found to be infected with Sars-Cov-2 when they are tested in the hospital.

But part of the increase in hospitalizations is real. And some regional hospital networks are under strain. The evidence is clear: the coronavirus is spreading faster in the United States than it has in months.

All by itself this fact should raise serious questions about how well masks prevent the transmission of the coronavirus. Health authorities have told Americans for six months to wear masks. We have listened. More of us are wearing masks more often than ever before. Yet the virus is spreading faster.

How can that be, if masks work?

6

The answer is that the evidence that face coverings do any good turns out to be even more porous than masks themselves.

Understanding why requires some background in the biology of viruses and the ways they spread.

Figuring out how Sars-Cov-2 – or any respiratory virus – jumps between people is very complicated. Figuring out if masks reduce transmission is even more so. Some of the language scientists use adds to the confusion in ways that make masks seem more effective than they are.

We know Sars-Cov-2 spreads mainly through the air. Transmission through touching "fomites" on contaminated surfaces is less common than was initially thought. Infected people exhale viral particles – virions – that are usually carried inside larger molecules made mostly of water and called "aerosols" or "droplets." People around the infected person inhale those aerosols or droplets and are exposed to the virus.

The distinction between an aerosol and a droplet is size: aerosols are smaller. But the word "droplet" doesn't mean what it seems to mean. It does *not* imply a raindrop-sized visible particle, like a mucus ball that a person with a cold might blow into a handkerchief.

An average raindrop is about 1/25th of an inch, or 1 millimeter – 1/1000th of a meter. Most people can't see objects smaller than about 0.1 millimeters without using a magnifying glass or microscope.

Viruses, aerosols, and droplets are measured on much smaller scales.

Below a millimeter, the next common unit of length is the micrometer or micron. A micron is 1/1000th of a millimeter, or 1/1,000,000th of a meter. The smallest object people can see – 0.1 millimeters – equals 100 microns.

When scientists talk about "droplets," they mean any exhaled particle more than 5 microns, 1/5000th of an inch, far too small for anyone to see unaided. Aerosols are even smaller – less than 5 microns.

The coronavirus itself is smaller still. For it, scientists use still another measure of length, the nanometer. 1 nanometer is 1/1000th of a micron. In other words, 1 meter equals one *billion* nanometers. An average-sized man is about 1,700,000,000 nanometers tall.

But a single virion of Sars-Cov-2 is about 60 to 140 nanometers, or 0.1 microns.

The different measurement scales can be confusing.

But the first takeaway is simple. Whatever masks do – or don't do – to protect us from the coronavirus is mostly *invisible*. Masks can obviously catch visible chunks of spit or phlegm, but the virus mostly travels on much smaller particles.

The second takeaway is also simple. All masks are not created equal, even if they all look more or less the same. For a mask to provide decent protection, it must be made of a material fine enough to catch nearly all of those tiny aerosols and droplets.

Such face coverings do exist.

Technically, they aren't called masks at all, but respirators.

Respirators must be certified as offering specific levels of protection before they're sold. In the United States, the most common models are called N95s. They have that name because manufacturers must prove they catch at least 95 percent of all particles of 300 nanometers – 0.3 microns. Many N95 masks prove even more effective than that standard in laboratory testing, blocking up to 99 percent of all but the smallest particles.

In contrast, standards for surgical masks are far less strict, and standards for homemade cloth masks don't exist. (Surgical masks are often light blue and made of three layers. The inside and outside are non-woven fabric, the middle a thin melted plastic layer, usually polypropylene. Cloth masks can be made of almost any fabric and can be one or multiple layers. Most Americans now seem to wear cloth masks in public, though surgical masks are also common.)

Further, unlike ordinary masks, N95 respirators are supposed to be "fit-tested." In other words, they're meant to attach tightly to the face of the person wearing them, with no gaps that allow unfiltered air between their edges and the skin. "The respirator must fit the user's face snugly (i.e., create a seal," the Centers for Disease Control wrote in an advisory about masks in March.

(https://blogs.cdc.gov/niosh-science-blog/2020/03/16/n95-preparedness/)

But ordinary masks are not fit-tested. Sometimes they are tied over the ear. More frequently they come with preattached loops. So ordinary masks start with two huge disadvantages compared to N95s. Their material offers less protection, *and* they don't fit as well.

But N95s are expensive, and even trained medical staff dislike wearing them for more than a few hours. As two doctors wrote in a commentary in August, "when worn properly, N95 masks are suffocating, uncomfortable, and difficult to tolerate for long durations."

(https://jamanetwork.com/journals/jamainternalmedicine/fullarticle/2769441)

As a practical matter, if civilians are going to wear face coverings, they will be standard cloth or surgical masks. But the limitations of those masks were well documented long before the coronavirus epidemic.

In 2009, four researchers examined how well surgical masks worked to filter small particles, those of 1 micron (1000 nanometers) or less. Their conclusion: badly.

In a paper called "Filtration Performance of FDA-Cleared Surgical Masks," the scientists tested five surgical mask brands. Four of the five masks allowed 15 percent or more of 100-nanometer (virus-sized) to 1 micron-sized particles through. Two of the five allowed more than half of those particles through.

Making matters worse, the authors believed their results actually overstated the real-world performance of the masks. They had sealed their masks to the "faces" of their mannikins with silicone. "A surgical mask user would be expected to get protection levels far less than that observed in this study, because a complete sealing of a surgical mask to a human face cannot be achieved," they wrote.

They concluded with a warning: "The wide variation in penetration levels for room air particles, which included particles in the same size range of viruses, confirms that **surgical masks should not be used for respiratory protection** [emphasis added]."

(https://www.ncbi.nlm.nih.gov/pmc/articles/PMC7357397/)

More recent studies have also found surgical masks were mostly ineffective compared to N95s.

One paper was published in August and focused on the question of whether expired N95s were still safe to use. On that issue, the researchers found good news. Long after their posted expiration dates, most N95s still worked.

But as part of the study, the researchers also checked the performance of surgical masks. And they used human subjects rather than mannikins, for a more realistic demonstration of the way masks fit.

The scientists found the surgical masks barely worked. Masks with ties filtered about 70 percent of small particles. Those with ear loops filtered less than 40 percent and often had "visible gaps between the face mask and the wearer."

(Dr. Michael Osterholm, an infectious disease expert, made the same point more graphically in a June podcast interview. Based on the pictures he saw of people wearing masks, about one person in four was wearing them wrongly, the equivalent "of fixing three of the five screen doors on your submarine." Rather than masks, Osterholm said he preferred to focus on encouraging people to stay at least six feet apart.[3])

The August paper makes clear that – if a shortage of new N95s forces them to choose – health-care workers should pick old N95s over new surgical masks. But the authors didn't explicitly say so in their conclusion, maybe because they were aware that *any* criticism of masks is off-limits in the coronavirus era.

---

[3] https://www.ama-assn.org/delivering-care/public-health/covid-19-s-first-wave-may-be-only-wave-no-pause)

Instead, they pointed out that their work offered "quantitative results... [for] evidence-based decisions."

In other words, *we're not going to tell you surgical masks don't work – you can read.*

(https://jamanetwork.com/article.aspx?doi=10.1001/jamainternmed.2020.4221)

What's true for surgical masks appears to be doubly true for homemade cloth masks, which generally filter even fewer small particles and are even *less* effective. The overall evidence is clear: Standard cloth and surgical masks offer next to no protection against virus-sized particles or small aerosols.

But maybe that failure doesn't matter. Can we be sure that the virus actually floats in particles that small?

Yes.

In a paper published in the November International Journal of Infectious Diseases, a team of researchers reported finding Sars-Cov-2 viral particles floating in the air of a hospital room. The virus they collected could reproduce in cell cultures – meaning it was "alive," not merely dead fragments of viral particles.

In their conclusion, the researchers explained:

> The public health implications are broad, particularly as current best practices for limiting the spread of COVID-19 center on social distancing, **wearing of face coverings while in proximity to others** [emphasis added] and hand washing. For aerosol-based transmission, measures such as physical distancing by 6 feet would not be helpful in an indoor setting,

provide a false sense of security, and lead to exposures and outbreaks.

Once again, the researchers didn't explicitly say that if physical distancing "would not be helpful" against aerosol-based transmission, *masks* also wouldn't be. Such is the pressure to encourage mask wearing.

(https://www.sciencedirect.com/science/article/pii/S1201971220307396)

The fact dormitories, prisons, ships, and other "congregate" settings can see very high rates of coronavirus infection – as high as 90 percent – also provides strong real-world evidence that Sars-Cov-2 spreads through tiny aerosol particles that stay in the air for long periods. Person-to-person transmission would be unlikely to spread the virus that quickly or effectively.

In one study of coronavirus transmission in a San Francisco homeless shelter, researchers found that they could track only four "close contacts" to the two original cases at the shelter, and 18 people in beds within six feet. But in testing only three to four days after the initial positive tests from the first two cases, 101 residents of the shelter tested positive. At the time, San Francisco had very low community transmission of Sars-Cov-2, so it is likely the residents were infected inside the shelter.

(https://www.ncbi.nlm.nih.gov/pmc/articles/PMC7454344/)

In fact, as early as February, Chinese health authorities warned that "aerosol transmission" was a major transmission route. They urged people to keep windows open.

(https://www.chinadaily.com.cn/a/202002/08/WS5e3e7d97a310128217275fc3.html)

The theoretical evidence that cloth and surgical masks do not protect their wearers is overwhelming. But we have even *stronger* evidence. It comes from real-world clinical trials of people wearing masks.

Medical proof comes in many different forms.

The weakest evidence comes from anecdotes based on one person's experience. Just because I didn't have an accident after driving drunk doesn't mean doing so is safe.

On the other hand, the gold standard of evidence comes from what scientists and physicians call randomized controlled trials. In those trials, researchers recruit people and split them into evenly matched groups. They then offer one group a certain treatment and another no treatment.

Suppose I believe a cholesterol-lowering drug called a statin can reduce heart disease. I give some of the people in my trial the statin and the rest a placebo pill that contains no medicine. When the trial is over, I check whether the people who took the statin had fewer heart attacks and strokes than the ones who received the placebo pill. If they did, I can assume the statin is responsible for the difference. In fact, companies and independent researchers have run many such trials and consistently found statins reduce heart disease. So if you have high cholesterol, your doctor will prescribe a statin.

But it's crucial to remember that even if I have reason to think a treatment will work, *unless I run the trial I don't know.* Drug companies spent billions of dollars on another kind of cholesterol-lowering medicine called a CETP inhibitor. But when they tested those drugs in clinical trials, they found deaths *rose.* They had to quit developing them.

Even a good idea can fail in practice, which is why the four most important words in medicine are *"First, do no harm."* For centuries, well-meaning physicians used techniques we find horrifying today, in part because they depended on anecdotal evidence and hope rather than hard data from clinical trials.

Anecdotes are on one end; clinical trial evidence is on the other. A huge variety of data exists between the two. Some is what scientists call pre-clinical, like "in vitro" studies on cells in laboratories, or animal research, or mechanistic studies designed to show how and why a treatment might work. All those studies should be viewed with caution. No one can be sure how lab results will translate into humans. Cancer researchers often joke that they've cured tumors many times – in mice.

Another form of evidence is real-world data in people that doesn't come out of a clinical trial.

For example, researchers might track whether people who have quit drinking are less likely to start again if they go to Alcoholics Anonymous meetings. Or they might try to figure out what's causing changes in even larger groups. Why have car accidents risen in one state but not another? We call this kind of work epidemiology – trying to measure and control diseases and dangerous behaviors in groups of people.

But this research has a huge caveat. Unless they set up the groups in advance, researchers cannot know if the people in the two groups were truly the same going in. So they can't be sure what has caused the changes they see.

In the AA example, maybe the people who went to AA meetings seem less likely to drink again *because they were so motivated to stop drinking that they went to meetings,* not because of any help the meetings themselves provide. Or maybe not – maybe the meetings actually work. (Addiction researchers have debated this issue for decades.)

Worse, as the groups get bigger and more diverse, researchers will have a harder and harder time figuring out what's really causing the changes.

Thus when we're trying to figure out whether a treatment actually works, the best evidence by far comes from clinical trials. Nothing else comes close.

And clinical trials consistently find that masks *don't* protect people from respiratory viruses.

In February, seven researchers in Hong Kong reviewed *all* the trials they could find that tested whether masks outside hospital settings protected their wearers against the flu. They found 10 studies that had been conducted since 1946. (The number is relatively small, given the importance of the question. The reason is that trials are expensive. Prescription drug companies, which pay for most of them, have no incentive to spend money figuring out if masks work.)

The researchers combined the results of the 10 trials into a single "meta-analysis" – a review that looks at each study and figures out what they say as a whole. Their conclusion – published in Emerging Infectious Diseases, a Centers for Disease Control journal – was straightforward:

> We **did not find evidence** that surgical-type face masks are effective in reducing laboratory-confirmed influenza transmission, either when worn by infected persons (source control) or by

persons in the general community to reduce their susceptibility. [Emphasis added]

(https://wwwnc.cdc.gov/eid/article/26/5/19-0994_article)

A trial published in 2015 on cloth and surgical masks used by healthcare workers in Vietnam reached an even more depressing conclusion. The study was the first randomized trial to examine the use of cloth masks, which healthcare workers in poorer countries commonly wear.

The researchers found healthcare workers who wore cloth masks were *more* likely to develop infections than those who wore surgical masks as well as a third control group who were not required to wear masks at all. The trial did not include N95 respirators, since respirators are uncommon in poorer countries and the researchers wanted to offer realistic alternatives.

But the researchers did put both masks and N95s through lab tests to see how easily particles penetrated them. They found that cloth masks stopped only 3 percent of particles, and medical masks stopped just over half. The N95s stopped 99.9 to 99.99 percent of particles.

In their discussion, the researchers wrote that the trial

> suggests HCWs [health-care workers] should not use cloth masks as protection against respiratory infection... the physical properties of a cloth mask, reuse, the frequency and effectiveness of cleaning, and increased moisture retention, may potentially increase the infection risk for HCWs.

(https://www.ncbi.nlm.nih.gov/pmc/articles/PMC4420971/)

Of course, none of these studies specifically looked at Sars-Cov-2, since they were all conducted before this year. They were also all relatively small.

If only we had a large randomized controlled trial that specifically examined whether masks protected their wearers from the coronavirus.

Now we do.

In a paper published on Nov. 18, Danish researchers reported on a trial that covered almost 5,000 people in Denmark in the spring. The trial was carefully designed and executed, with half the participants told to wear high-quality surgical masks and provided 50 for free. The other half were not asked to wear masks. Participants were followed for a month to see if they had been infected with Sars-Cov-2.

Within the month, 53 people in the maskless group had been infected, compared to 42 who wore masks. The difference was indistinguishable from chance, and suggested masks might really cause anywhere from a 46 percent decrease to a 23 percent *increase* in infections among their wearers.

The reason for the failure was not that people in the masked group didn't follow the rules, either. When they looked at only at participants who always wore masks, the researchers found an even smaller difference. Mask wearing "did not reduce, at conventional levels of statistical significance, the incidence of Sars-Cov-2 infection," the authors wrote in their discussion.

(https://www.acpjournals.org/doi/10.7326/M20-6817)

Unless future large randomized controlled trials find different results, the Danish mask study essentially should end the debate if surgical masks protect people who wear them outside hospitals.

As physicians and infectious disease professionals largely agreed until April, the answer is that they don't. Anyone who says otherwise, for whatever reason, is being untruthful – and as of Nov. 10, that group, unfortunately, includes the Centers for Disease Control.

7

But what about the second part of the promise mask advocates make: that my mask protects *you*, while yours protects *me*?

And what about the mandates that flow out of that promise – that for us to protect each other, we *all* must wear masks, even if we are not showing symptoms of Covid?

Those questions turn out to be even *more* complicated than the one of whether masks protect their wearers. For the "my mask protects you" theory to be true and universal mask mandates to make sense, several different and highly technical questions must align. Those include:

The size of the particles people exhale;

The filtration characteristics of ordinary cloth and surgical masks;

Whether people are wearing masks properly;

The number of viral particles needed to cause an infection;

The relative risk of infection inside and outside and how well the virus can survive in sunlight or harsh conditions;

The question of whether people who are infected with Covid but not showing symptoms can have sufficient viral loads to infect other people.

We don't have precise answers to all of those questions. But the answers we do have tend not to support the logic behind source control – "my mask protects you."

The theory is essentially as follows: infected people exhale the virus in both droplets and aerosols, large and small particles. A mask, even a cloth mask, can catch droplets and thus reduce the total amount of virus a person is exhaling. Plus, because large particles tend to fall to the ground quickly, masks are even *more* important when two people are close together. The reason is in that case the mask might provide some protection to the wearer, too – because it will catch droplets that the person would otherwise inhale before they hit the ground.

Intuitively, the idea makes sense. But the details are crucial.

For example, if most particles people exhale are very small, catching larger particles may not matter much. Measuring the exact size of the particles in people's breath is technically challenging. But in 2009 researchers did so. What they found is not good for mask advocates. The vast majority of particles in exhaled breath are tiny, smaller than a micron.

In the paper, called "Size distribution and sites of origin of droplets expelled from the human respiratory tract during expiratory activities," the researchers reported:

> The majority of droplets from human expiratory activities are very small, being in low micrometer and high sub-micrometer ranges. Where Papineni and Rosenthal [an earlier study] found that 80–90% of droplets were smaller than 1 μm [micron], the current study agrees, showing that these smallest particles are located within an aerosol mode, centered in the range 0.1–1 μm.

(https://www.sciencedirect.com/science/article/pii/S00218502 08002036)

In basic terms, masks have almost no chance of catching most of the particles we exhale.

Of course, if larger droplets happen to hold most Sars-Cov-2 virions, then maybe masks can help even if they don't do much good against smaller particles. For many years, scientists believed large droplets *did* hold most viral particles – in part because they simply have much more room. Imagine a marble in a box – if the box is a foot on each side, it can hold the marble easily, but if it is only an inch, the marble will have to drop in perfectly.

But just as researchers can now determine the size of the particles that people exhale, they now know which particles hold virions. Again, the answer is not good for the source control theory.

In a remarkable paper published in the September 2020 issue of The Lancet: Respiratory Medicine, Dr. Kevin P. Fennelly – a pulmonologist at the National Heart, Lung, and Blood Institute – debunked the view that larger droplets are responsible for most viral transmission. Fennelly wrote:

> Current infection control policies are based on the premise that most respiratory infections are transmitted by large respiratory droplets—ie, larger than 5 μm [microns] — produced by coughing and sneezing...

Unfortunately, that premise is wrong, Fennelly explained.

Studies "that included methods to measure particle sizes have consistently found pathogens in small particles (i.e. under 5 microns)." A study of influenza patients found about two-thirds of all the virus was contained in particles under 4 microns.

Other researchers found that particles under 5 microns contained 9 times as much flu virus as larger particles. (That paper did show surgical masks cut the amount of virus found in smaller particles – a point for "my mask protects you" – but by far less than they reduced the virus in larger particles.)

"There is no evidence that some pathogens are carried only in large droplets," Fennelly wrote. Even the fact that risk rose when people were close together didn't provide much evidence for the droplet theory. Small particles also had a higher risk of infecting people at short distances.

Making matters worse, some pathogens are *more* dangerous when they spread via smaller particles, probably because smaller particles penetrate more deeply into the lungs than larger ones. Fennelly noted a breakthrough 1953 paper on anthrax that showed that single bacterial spore of about one micron was significantly more lethal than larger clumps of spores.

Fennelly did not go so far as to call masks useless – a near impossibility in the current environment – but he was lukewarm at best on their value to protect other people even in the most obvious case, when they are worn by symptomatic patients in hospitals. "Masking of patients can help to partly reduce infectious aerosol exposures to health-care workers, but are not a substitute for physical distancing and other infection control measures."

Instead, he called for a focus on improving ventilation as well as "air disinfection with ultraviolet germicidal irradiation," especially for nursing homes, where so many Covid deaths have occurred.

(https://www.thelancet.com/journals/lanres/article/PIIS2213-2600(20)30323-4/fulltext)

Further, even if masks do keep people from exhaling enough large particles to reduce the amount of virus around them substantially, and even if large and small particles are equally dangerous, and even if people wear masks properly –

Forcing everyone to wear masks will matter very little unless asymptomatic people spread the coronavirus in large numbers. Everyone agrees people who are symptomatic with a fever or cough should stay home or wear a mask if they must go out. If only sick people are wearing masks, face coverings may function as a public signal: *I don't feel well, stay away.*

But the *point* of universal mask mandates is to force people who do not feel sick to wear masks anyway, on the theory that people without symptoms can also spread the virus.

Like practically every other part of the "my mask protects you" theory, this aspect is unproven. Worse – like the advice around general lockdowns, which were never recommended before March – it has become highly politicized. Scientists including Anthony Fauci have reversed course on the likelihood of asymptomatic transmission. At a press conference in January, Fauci could not have been clearer. Asymptomatic transmission was not a threat:

> The one thing historically people need to realize is that even if there is some asymptomatic transmission, in all the history of respiratory-borne viruses of any type, asymptomatic transmission has never been the driver of outbreaks. The driver of outbreaks is always a symptomatic person. Even if there's a rare asymptomatic person that might transmit, an epidemic is not driven by asymptomatic carriers.

At a press conference on June 8, a senior World Health Organization scientist also said people almost never transmitted the coronavirus if they did not have at least mild symptoms. In response to a question about asymptomatic transmission, Maria Van Kerkhove, an epidemiologist and the "technical lead" for WHO's Covid-19 response team, said:

> We have a number of reports from countries who are doing very detailed contact tracing. They're following asymptomatic cases, they're following contacts and they're not finding secondary transmission onward. It's very rare.

People who were reported to be asymptomatic generally had at least mild disease, like a low fever or cough, Van Kerkhove said.

(https://www.who.int/docs/default-source/coronaviruse/transcripts/who-audio-emergencies-coronavirus-press-conference-08jun2020.pdf?sfvrsn=f6fd460a_0)

The relative lack of asymptomatic transmission shouldn't be surprising, for the coronavirus or any respiratory illness, because *symptoms and severity of illness usually rise with viral load.* As early as March, Chinese researchers reported that "our data indicate that... patients with severe Covid-19 tend to have a high viral load and a long shedding period." An August study reached a similar conclusion.

(https://www.thelancet.com/journals/laninf/article/PIIS1473-3099(20)30232-2/fulltext)

Of course, some people can show no symptoms even when testing reveals they have relatively high levels of the virus.

Other studies have shown no or a small overall difference in viral loads between symptomatic and asymptomatic patients. And computer modeling suggests that up to 40 percent of infections could come from asymptomatic cases.

But when real-world contact tracers tried to find actual evidence of asymptomatic spread of Sars-Cov-2, they are basically unable to do so. In July, the WHO noted that four studies had showed that "between 0% and 2.2% of people with asymptomatic infection infected anyone else."

(https://www.who.int/news-room/commentaries/detail/transmission-of-sars-cov-2-implications-for-infection-prevention-precautions)

The most stunning example of this came from a city-wide screening for Sars-Cov-2 in May in Wuhan, China, where the virus apparently originated. Researchers tried to test *everyone* in Wuhan. They nearly succeeded, carrying out almost 10 million tests. They found 303 people who tested positive for the virus. All 303 cases were asymptomatic. The scientists then traced 1174 close contacts of those people – and found not one had been infected. "There was no evidence of transmission from asymptomatic positive persons," they wrote.

(https://www.nature.com/articles/s41467-020-19802-w)

But the media and other public health experts immediately pushed back on Van Kerkhove's accidental honesty in the June 8 press conference. Why? Because the threat of asymptomatic transmission is critical to the argument for universal mask mandates.

If people without symptoms are very unlikely to transmit Sars-Cov-2 to others, why make them wear masks at all? The evidence is overwhelming that surgical or cloth masks don't protect their wearers, so whom exactly are the masks protecting?

Within 48 hours, Van Kerkhove and the WHO were forced to walk back their statement, at least partially. The organization tried to distinguish between "asymptomatic" and "presymptomatic" carriers – people who had just been infected and were about to get sick but hadn't yet. Those presymptomatic carriers might have a short window where they were infectious.

In reality, though Van Kerkhove's statement was in keeping with the WHO's views about asymptomatic transmission and masks. On June 5, the organization had released a statement entitled "Advice on the use of masks in the context of Covid-19." The paper ran 16 pages and included 80 footnotes and this stunning statement:

> At the present time, the widespread use of masks by healthy people in the community setting **is not yet supported by high quality or direct scientific evidence** and there are potential benefits and harms to consider. [emphasis added]

(https://www.who.int/publications/i/item/advice-on-the-use-of-masks-in-the-community-during-home-care-and-in-healthcare-settings-in-the-context-of-the-novel-coronavirus-(2019-ncov)-outbreak)

The WHO then managed to choke out the weakest possible recommendation for mask use by healthy people: "**In areas of community transmission, governments should encourage the general public to wear masks in specific situations and settings.**"

How many caveats did WHO put on this supposed recommendation?

In a table, the paper explained that – for example – people working in countries with "limited or no capacity to implement other containment measures such as physical distancing [and] contact tracing" might "be encouraged" to wear non-medical masks. The reason: "**potential benefit** of source control." [emphasis added]

Just why was the WHO so lukewarm on wearing masks?

Though it runs to billions of dollars a year, the cost of forcing healthy adults to wear disposable surgical masks will be relatively minor for wealthy countries. And cloth masks are easy to clean in places that have access to clean water. In poor countries the calculus is different. Making people wear cloth masks that cannot be easily cleaned or spend a significant part of their income on disposable ones is much harder to justify if masks don't work.

The WHO said as much in the report, saying governments should consider "availability and costs of masks, access to clean water to wash non-medical masks, and ability of mask wearers to tolerate adverse effects of wearing a mask."

The science around masks and mask mandates has become deeply politicized since April.

That's why two Canadian arbitration decisions about masks from 2015 and 2018 – before face coverings became so totemic that people who didn't wear them risked being called sociopaths – are highly instructive.

The decisions arose from efforts by hospitals in the Canadian province of Ontario to force nurses to be vaccinated against influenza. The hospitals could not contractually make nurses take the vaccine.

Instead they decreed that any nurse who refused would instead be required to wear a surgical mask while working. Crucially, the hospitals were mainly concerned with using masks for "source control" – protecting *patients* from nurses who might be spreading the flu before they had symptoms.

In December 2013 the nurses' union filed a grievance against the policy. The case went to a neutral arbitrator, James Hayes. He heard thousands of pages of testimony from six expert witnesses, consulted 249 exhibits, and read more than 100 scientific papers.

In September 2015, Hayes issued a 136-page ruling saying hospitals could not make nurses wear masks. The "scientific evidence said to support the [mask mandate] on patient safety grounds is insufficient," he wrote.

Even the theory that masks could prevent droplet transmission was unproven, Hayes found:

> At best, there appears to be limited evidence of what to a layperson may seem obvious: a mask may prevent the transmission of large droplets. Two literature reviews refer specifically to "limited data" and to "the limited evidence base supporting the efficacy and effectiveness of face masks to reduce influenza virus transmission."

He went on to quote one of the experts the nurses offered:

> Coughing, sneezing and talking produce a wide range of particle sizes, all of which can be

infectious. The smaller-sized particles will easily bypass the filter and facepiece of a surgical mask—and are likely to remain airborne for long periods of time.

Later in the report, Hayes noted that even the experts the hospitals had offered agreed that "there is limited evidence on the significant point of the utility of masks in reducing transmission risk."

In addition, wearing masks for long periods came with downsides, the nurses' experts told Hayes. Masks were uncomfortable, became moist, and could cause skin irritation. (One referred to a "grunge factor.")

So Hayes struck down the requirement, finding that even in hospitals – where masks are likely far *more* useful than other settings, given that they are filled with vulnerable patients and regularly have outbreaks of respiratory illness – the evidence did not support for mask mandates for healthy adults.

(https://www.canlii.org/en/on/onla/doc/2015/2015canlii62106 /2015canlii62106.pdf)

The fight didn't end there. Some hospitals kept trying to make nurses wear masks. The nurses objected again. Again they won.

In a September 6, 2018 decision, arbitrator William Kaplan agreed with Hayes's ruling. In fact, Kaplan went further than Hayes, calling the evidence in favor of mask mandates "insufficient, inadequate, and completely unpersuasive." Later in his ruling, he wrote:

> The preponderance of the masking evidence is compelling – surgical and procedural masks are extremely limited in terms of source control:

they do not prevent the transmission of the
influenza virus.

(https://www.ona.org/wp-
content/uploads/ona_kaplanarbitrationdecision_vac
cinateormask_stmichaelsoha_20180906.pdf)

These arbitrators were not anti-mask. They were chosen for
their neutrality. But both looked at the evidence and reached
the same conclusion.

The decisions came in the context of the flu, not the
coronavirus. But all the evidence we have suggests that both
viruses, which are roughly the same size, are transmitted in the
same way.

The theoretical evidence lines up nearly as strongly against the
idea that "my mask protects you" as it does against "my mask
protects me."

What about the real-world evidence?

Unfortunately, we do not currently have a study as definitive as
the Danish mask trial for the source control theory. Such a trial
would be very hard to run – it would require something like
picking two similarly sized *cities* and requiring every healthy
person in one to wear masks for a month or more while banning
everyone in the other from doing so.

In the absence of such a trial, mask advocates have pointed to a
more or less random series of case reports and observational
data. For example, they have pointed to a CDC report showing
two coronavirus-infected hairdressers in Missouri who wore
masks did *not* infect 139 clients.

(https://www.cdc.gov/mmwr/volumes/69/wr/mm6928e2.htm)

The problem is that in the absence of other facts, we cannot know if the masks were the reason the hairdressers didn't infect their clients. Maybe the salon had good ventilation. Maybe the hairdressers happened not to be very infectious, since contact tracing studies show many people with Covid do not infect other people, while a small number of people appear to be so-called "super-spreaders."

Public health advocates also point to reports showing individual counties with mask mandates appeared to have slower growth in transmission rates than neighboring counties that did not. For example, a CDC report about the state of Kansas claimed that growth in positive tests was far lower in counties with mask mandates than those without.

(https://www.cdc.gov/mmwr/volumes/69/wr/mm6947e2.htm)

But this Kansas data is also much weaker than it appears at first. We don't know whether the rules translated into a major or even minor difference in mask use. More importantly, at the end of the period the CDC reviewed, the counties with mask mandates actually still had *higher* overall rates of Covid than those without.

Many, many other observational datapoints suggest that mask mandates have made no difference to the spread of Sars-Cov-2. Florida ended statewide mask mandates in late September, for example. But in the two months since, the state has had significantly slower growth in positive tests than the United States as a whole.

On a national basis, masks appear to have made even less difference. The United States is not alone in seeing huge spikes in positive Covid tests despite mask mandates and high levels of mask use. Most of Europe has had the same trend.

Epidemiologists agree that when clinical trials are impossible, real-world evidence must be nearly overwhelming to reach anything like the same level of proof. The best example comes with tobacco and lung cancer. Running a clinical trial to examine whether tobacco causes cancer would be both impossible and unethical. But heavy cigarette smokers develop lung cancer at rates 20 times those of nonsmokers – a difference that cannot be explained for any other reason. Even so, doctors and scientists argued for decades over potential other explanations before rejecting them.

In the case of the source control theory for masks, the real-world evidence is somewhere between weak and nonexistent. Yet instead of decades, public health authorities changed their collective mind on masks nearly overnight.

Meanwhile, though we don't have anything as good as the Danish study for source control, we do have the results of one real-world trial that touches on "my mask protects you." It was short, but well-run – and it too offers no joy to mask advocates.

This year, more than 3,000 Marine recruits participated in a two-week quarantine that included cloth mask wearing, social distancing, and daily temperature and symptom checks. They lived on a closed college campus which they could not leave. They did not even have access to "personal electronics and other items that might contribute to surface transmission."

Yet at the end of the quarantine, almost 2 percent of the Marines tested positive for the coronavirus – even in a group of Marines who were tested when the quarantine started to remove anyone who was already infected.

(https://www.nejm.org/doi/full/10.1056/NEJMoa2029717)

The study does not *prove* masks don't work as source control. Perhaps the Marines would have been infected at much higher rate if they had not been wearing face coverings. But an infection rate of 1 percent per week is hardly evidence masks work, especially given the many other protective measures the recruits used.

Yet despite the evidence that masks are of extremely marginal benefit at most for source control, public health authorities continue to insist on them.

The most obvious reasons are not medical but political.

The "good" reason is that masks are a visible totem that we are all working together against the coronavirus. We cannot all be physicians or nurses, but as they work to save lives, we all can sacrifice in this small way.

As Anthony Fauci said at a press conference in May, "It's not 100 percent effective. I mean, it's sort of respect for another person, and have that person respect you." He added that he wears masks "because I want to make it be a symbol for people to see that that's the kind of thing you should be doing."

(https://www.politico.com/news/2020/05/27/fauci-wears-mask-as-symbol-of-good-behavior-283847)

Of course, encouraging people to take actions that are (supposedly) symbolically valuable is different than *forcing* them. I may want to wear a pink pin to show I care about beating breast cancer, but Governor Cuomo can't make me.

At least I don't think he can, though I'm not so sure anymore.

The not-so-good reason is that making people wear masks frightens them. Frightens *us*. Masks are warnings none of us can escape. This virus is different. This virus is dangerous. This virus is *not* the flu. We had better hunker down until a vaccine is ready to save us all.

But the worst reason of all is that mask mandates appear to be an effort by governments to find out what restrictions on their civil liberties people will accept on the thinnest possible evidence. They are the not-so-thin edge of the wedge. Today, we must wear masks. Tomorrow we'll need negative Covid tests to travel between countries. Or vaccines to go to work.

I wish masks worked. I wish we didn't have to fight about them.

But they don't.

And we do.